GREEN & NATURAL

Acne & Seborrhea Care Recipes

GREEN & NATURAL
Acne & Seborrhea Care Recipes

Copyright 2011

L. Pippen

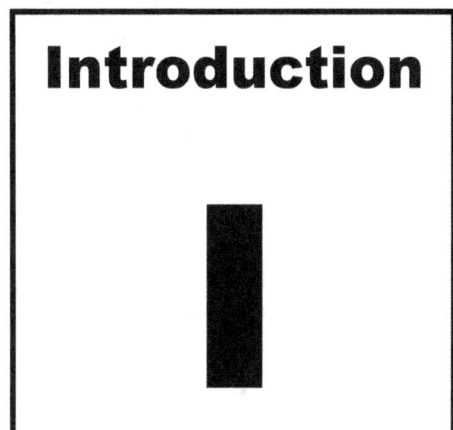

Introduction

Acne is a common skin condition that causes whiteheads, blackheads, cystitis, or seborrhea. Acne can occur for a variety of reasons. The most common cause of acne is a clogged follicle or pore. When glands produce too much oil, pores can become blocked with dirt, bacteria and old skin cells. The blockage is the most common cause of acne.

Acne can appear in different ways on different people. Common acne can appear as red, scaly skin known as seborrhea, as black or white-headed pustules, and as inflamed, red bumps that may produce scarring.

A white head happens when trapped sebum and bacteria stay just below the surface of the skin. The whitehead may appear on the surface as a white, raised spot. Some whiteheads are so small that they are nearly invisible while others may grow engorged to the point where they are very noticeable.

A blackhead occurs when the pore opens to the surface of the skin and sebum oxidizes. When sebum oxidizes, it turns a brown or black color. A blackhead is not dirt and cannot be washed away. A blackhead may be more difficult to treat because it could take a long time for all of the oxidized sebum to drain from the surface of the skin.

Both whiteheads and blackheads may release their contents by "popping". While this does speed the healing of that particular pimple, you should not pop it yourself. Rupturing a pimple can increase the risk of inflammatory acne and actually make the condition worse instead of better.

Inflammatory acne occurs if there is a break in the skin that causes white blood cells to make their way to the surface. This reaction creates inflammation and redness in the area surrounding the pimple. A nodule or large papule can form and is most frequently the cause of long-term scarring.

Scarring is a result of the inflammation that occurs within the skin when acne is present. The most common scar is actually created by the wound trying to heal itself. The wound puts too much collagen in one particular area. These scars tend to cause an indentation in the skin's surface.

Another acne related long-term mark often termed as a type of scarring, is a pigmentation scar. Pigmentation scars often occur because a nodule lying under the skin causes surface discoloration. These pigmentation scars often fade with time but may last forever if they are not treated.

Acne is most common in people during the pubescent years but it can happen to anyone, at any age. The most common cause of acne appears to be genetic, but some environmental factors and life choices can also aggravate acne.

Acne can appear on any part of your body and is found most heavily on the areas that have the highest number of sebaceous follicles. Acne is most commonly found on the face, shoulders, and buttocks.

There are many natural treatments & preventatives you can try to help reduce or even stop your acne outbreaks. Acne is very specific to each individual so you should start by considering your lifestyle and potential acne triggers. Each person may have one or more triggers that need to be corrected before the acne outbreaks can be stopped.

Acne outbreaks are most frequently caused by incomplete or incorrect cleaning of the skin. This results in blockages of the follicles or pores.

Hormonal changes can also cause acne outbreaks. These changes occur most often in puberty but may also be related to menstruation, menopause, and medications. During times of high hormonal fluctuations, follicular glands tend to grow larger and make more sebum. Sebum is the body's natural oil. Some individuals may develop seborrhea instead of acne in later life.

Increased stress or other psychological triggers may cause acne outbreaks. The exact mechanism that links stress to acne outbreaks is not clearly understood but may have a relationship to the hormonal changes caused by stress.

Bacterial infections may contribute to the severity of acne. Keeping the skin clean and resisting creating open wounds by popping blackheads or whiteheads can help to minimize the likelihood of infections.

A diet that is high in sugars, salt, or grease may be associated with acne outbreaks. The potential link between diet & acne outbreaks is controversial and additional research is necessary to determine how diet may affect acne.

You may be able to combat the severity of acne outbreaks by making some simple lifestyle changes.

You should always cleanse your skin & hair with a mild, non-drying soap product to ensure that you have removed all dirt, oils, and makeup. You may need to wash more than one time a day to keep the skin clean and clear. The formulas contained in this recipe book and the alternative ingredients will give you a wide range of options that you might use to keep your skin clean, hydrated, and acne free.

You should find a relaxation technique that helps to lower the hormonal changes related to stress and anxiety. While you cannot affect the hormonal changes that are a natural part of growing older, you can minimize the effect that stress and anxiety have on your life by learning a meditation or relaxation technique that works well for you.

You should spend some time logging the items in your diet to see if you can locate a link between certain types of food products and acne outbreaks. There is some controversy over whether diet really increases the severity of acne and additional research is constantly being undertaken to confirm or rule out food as a cause. In the meantime, you can conduct your own personal research by logging your dietary intake and outbreaks to see if there is a personal link for you.

Once you have located the potential triggers of outbreaks for your personal situation, you will have a better idea of how to treat and even prevent future outbreaks.

The recipes in this book have been compiled to help treat the symptoms of acne outbreaks in individuals close to me. You can try the recipes as they are written, or refer to the ingredient guide in the back of the recipe book to see if an alternative ingredient might work better for you. Remember, each person will have a slightly different situation including triggers, skin type, environment, and genetic history. You should experiment to find the perfect solution for you!

Natural care is about more than just using nature to solve a problem. Natural care is about CUSTOMIZING nature to solve your personal problem!

Soaps

Perhaps the most basic product in your daily personal care ritual is soap. Before you can use any other product in your regimen the area you are treating must be clean. People sometimes overlook the importance of using the correct soap.

Consider that soap is the first item, and often the last, that you use each day. People often spend the rest of the day using products to counteract the effects of the soap that they have chosen. Using the correct soap can either harm or enhance the results of the rest of your products.

Some people prefer soft soap and that is my favorite method for cleaning my face. Other people prefer a harder soap especially for body care.

Before deciding which soap recipe to try, you should understand the basics of skin and skin care. Many factors can affect the condition and appearance of skin. No soap or other product can replace simple daily care in your activities. Skin is the largest organ you have and perhaps the most important in that it protects every other part of you from environmental factors. Of course, skin is also very important because it is the first thing most people will notice about you.

People have been creating soaps for generations. The best way to achieve perfection in your soap-making endeavor is to keep experimenting to determine which soap works best with your skin, lifestyle, and climate. This chapter outlines the creation of the most common types of soap that you can customize to suit your needs. I have also included a few of my favorite soap customizations for you to use as a starting point. Remember to experiment – most of the ingredients in soap making are extremely cost effective and easy to locate. You can customize a different soap for each member of your family and then produce these a few times a year for less than you would commonly pay for a decent quality, but generic soap in the stores.

Soap recipes are often the most difficult for people to follow. Soap requires more time and effort than most of the other products included in this book. Do not be discouraged by the processes described since soap is a common item that has been successfully created by individuals for generations. To create exceptional soaps you just need to practice and perfect your skills. You will also need some dedicated equipment to create soap. You can easily find these items in specialty craft stores or often in an all-in-one retail chain. Some stores even carry kits that contain most of the key equipment in one package.

Cleansing is one of the best places that you can spend time experimenting and customizing the recipes to suit your needs. The better customized your cleansing regimen is to your particular skin type, lifestyle, and needs the better your appearance will be.

You may need to use different cleansers on different parts of your skin. Facial acne tends to be a slightly different problem than back acne and will need different treatments and preventatives. You should consider the underlying cause of the acne, sensitivity of the areas, and personal application preferences before selecting recipes to try.

Regardless of the recipes you choose to try it is always recommended that you test sample the products on a sensitive area such as your wrist to ensure that you do not have unexpected reactions before applying them to your skin. This is not a fail proof method of ensuring that the products are correct for you but it can often provide a warning of a negative reaction.

You should also look up each ingredient in the ingredient listing to determine potential side effects of using any natural product. Natural products contain medicinal qualities and you need to ensure that each inclusion is safe and effective for your personal needs.

Basic Supplies

Thermometer –   Successful soap making depends heavily on temperature.

The base components like lye, borax, and fat must be heated to a particular temperature and then cooled to become soap.

A good method of ensuring that you reach the proper temperatures is to buy a decent candy thermometer for use in your soap making.

The thermometer should be used only for one particular type of soap and should be dedicated only to soap making. If you decide to experiment with soaps that have a variety of bases you will want to obtain a few thermometers since using the same thermometer for lye that you use for fat bases can throw off the results of your soap-making endeavor.

Thermometers can be found in most craft stores or in the cooking section of your grocery store. The thermometer you select does not need to be the most advanced or expensive model available. A simple, cost-effective thermometer will work just fine for these recipes.

Cooking Pot -   You will need a glass or steel pot for heating and mixing.

You should have a dedicated mixing container for your soap making endeavors. While most of the ingredients in soap are safe, you would not want to eat out of the same pan you just used for boiling lye. You also want to be careful not to transfer foods, spices, and other cooking matter into your soap. These can irritate or worsen the conditions you are trying to treat.

It is important not to use aluminum or iron pots and pans when creating soap. The metal in these pots can react with the ingredients of the soap. A basic steel or enamel-coated pot works best and is often the most cost-effective purchase. You can find these in most retail chain stores.

Wooden Utensils - You will want to purchase a set of wooden utensils for soap making.

You should get a set of utensils that will be dedicated for use only with your product recipes. Again, these utensils should not be used for general cooking.

The type of utensils that have longer handles work well when making soap. You will need to stir deep into your cooking pots to ensure all the ingredients are well mixed and a longer handle makes it easier to stir and to prevent accidental contact between the ingredients and your hands.

Wooden utensils are heat resistant, will hold up better under some of the stronger ingredients you may choose to use, and will usually not cause an adverse reaction. You should not use metal utensils when making soap.

Gloves –   You will want to use a pair of kitchen gloves to protect your hands from the ingredients used in soap making.

You will use the final product of your soap making process on your skin, but the core ingredients can cause irritation or even burns before they are diluted into the recipe. Using a pair of kitchen gloves is the best practice during your soap making. These will protect your hands from inadvertent splashing and prevent problems that will then need to be treated using a different recipe.

Soap Molds -   You will need a mold or container to hold your completed soap during the hardening stage.

These recipes will often finish as a cake of soap. To achieve these perfectly formed cakes, you will need to use a mold. There are many molds available in specialty craft stores as well as at retail chain stores. Soap making has gained popularity in the last few years, making these products easier to find than ever before. You can find molds ranging from the very basic cake soap style to the more specialized styles that will suit your décor.

If you are using your soap yourself, you might not be as concerned with achieving the perfect appearance as you are with usefulness. You do not need to purchase specialized soap molds. Many items found in your house can be used as a mold.

You can use old baking pans such as muffin pans, cookie cutters, or bread pans as soap molds. You can even make your own mold out of old cardboard boxes. Almost any container that can withstand the heat of the liquid soap and will hold the liquid soap in place while it hardens will work as a mold.

Soap Making Dos!

When making soap, you must work in a well-ventilated area. Liquid and heated forms of some ingredients included in the soap making process can create fumes that may be harmful if inhaled.

Always wear gloves and other protective clothing when making soap since lye and other ingredients can burn or irritate the skin.

Always use COLD Distilled Water when mixing lye solutions.

Pour the lye mixture into the fat mixture not the other way around.

Keep solvents like vinegar nearby to neutralize the effect of the ingredients if they should touch the skin.

Remember that lye is a poison and should always be kept in a safe place.

Only create heated soap mixtures when you can be sure that you will not be distracted. Some of the ingredients and the heat processes involved in soap making can be dangerous. In addition, the recipes included in this chapter require a fine attention to detail to ensure success in your soap-making endeavor.

Beeswax Soap

Beeswax soap is become more popular for all types of treatments and especially for acne care. The natural healing and antibacterial properties of beeswax make it a soap option with a wide range of uses. Beeswax also leaves a thin protective coating on the skin making it one of the better quality soaps for those with sensitive or dry skin.

Creating this soap is sometimes a bit more expensive than the other forms since beeswax can be more costly. Check with your health food stores or a beekeeping compound in your area to find the best price on beeswax.

The following recipe will make approximately 1 bar of soap. You can enlarge it if you want to make a bigger batch.

Heat 1/3 cup of your favorite vegetable-based oil.

Review the optional ingredient list to determine which oil will provide the most beneficial effect for your needs.

Add 4 tsp. grated beeswax to the oils and heat until melted.

The mixture will be approximately 90 degrees.

While your oils are heating, dissolve 2 tsp. lye in 1/3 cup cold Distilled Water.

Remember to wear protective gloves and clothing when working with lye since lye can burn your skin.

Store your unused lye granules in a safe place since lye is a poison.

Remove your oil mixture from the heat and allow it to allow cool slightly to approximately 70 degrees.

You will probably want to customize the soap mixture with the ingredients that best meet your particular needs. The recipes on the following pages will give you some starter ideas. The ingredient list included in this books glossary will give you a much more comprehensive idea of which additives will work best for you.

While I do use additives that can prove beneficial for certain conditions, I typically do not add color or fragrance to any product designed for damaged or sensitive skin because additives can cause the irritation to worsen. If you prefer something other than the natural color or scent, you can add your favorite colorant, essential oils or herbs to the mixture.

Slowly pour the lye solution into the oil mixture.

Stir the mixture gently but well to ensure that all of the ingredients are blended.

If the soap mixture does not thicken within 30 minutes or if there is a greasy layer on the top of the mixture it may be too warm.

Set the container in a pan of cool Distilled Water.

Continue stirring, making sure to stir the sides and bottom of the pan to ensure an even mix.

The mixture will become thicker taking on the consistency of syrup.

If the soap mixture is too lumpy, it may be too cold. If this occurs, reverse the above process.

Sit the mixture in a pan of warm Distilled Water stirring until the lumps dissolve. You may need to replace the warm Distilled Water more than once until the mixture is heated to the correct temperature for effective blending.

Remember that everyone's skin reacts differently. You should test the products on a less sensitive area before using them. You should also remember that even natural products have side effects. The appendix gives the most common expected benefits and results of these ingredients. You should review these entries before trying any recipe.

Pour the thickened mixture into your molds, cover, and keep it in a warm place for at least 2 days. This helps to keep the mixture from separating.

Once the soap has set, remove the finished soap from the molds and cut it into bars.

Place the soap in a dry area until you are ready to use it.

Castile Soap

A nice soap base alternative to traditional bars is castile soap. To be castile soap the mixture must contain at least 40% olive oil. You can purchase ready-made castile soap and then customize the mixture to suit your needs or you may create castile soap at home.

This soap is especially mild and gentle making it a good selection for damaged or irritated skin. Castile soap is a versatile soap, you can even use the same castile soap products to wash your hair as you use for the rest of your body. You should test castile soap on a smaller area before using it in treatments for acne since the oils may cause extra irritation in some people.

The following recipe will yield the equivalent of 1 bar of soap. You can increase the recipe if you want to make a larger batch.

Heat 1/3 cup of olive oil to approximately 80 degrees Fahrenheit.

While the oil is heating, dissolve 2 tsp. lye granules in 1/3 cup cold Distilled Water.

Remember to wear protective gloves and clothing when working with lye since lye can burn your skin. Store your unused lye granules in a safe place because lye is a poison.

Remove your oil mixture from the heat and allow it to cool slightly to approximately 70 degrees.

You will probably want to customize the soap mixture with the ingredients that best meet your particular needs. The recipes on the following pages will give you some starter ideas. The ingredient list included in this books glossary will give you a much more comprehensive idea of which additives will work best for you.

While I do use additives that can prove beneficial for certain conditions, I typically do not add color or fragrance to any product designed for damaged or sensitive skin because additives can cause the irritation to worsen. If you prefer something other than the natural color or scent, you can add your favorite colorant, essential oils or herbs to the mixture.

Slowly pour the lye solution into the oil mixture.

Stir the mixture gently but well to ensure that all of the ingredients are well blended.

Allow the mixture to cool before placing it in a dispenser jar. If you want to convert liquid castile soap to a bar product, you will add a thickening agent and emulsifier and pour the finished mixture into molds as you would with any bar soap.

Remember that everyone's skin reacts differently. You should test the products on a less sensitive area before using them. You should also remember that even natural products have side effects. The appendix gives the most common expected benefits and results of these ingredients. You should review these entries before trying any recipe.

Coconut Oil Soap

Coconut oil is an excellent skin protectant and is one of the nicest natural foaming products that you can find to use in the soap making process

The following recipe will yield approximately 1 bar of soap. You can increase the recipe if you want a bigger batch.

Heat 3 teaspoons of coconut oil and ¼ cup vegetable-based oil on low heat to approximately 75 degrees Fahrenheit.

While the mixture is heating, dissolve 2 tsp. lye granules in 1/3 cup cold Distilled Water.

Remember to wear protective gloves and clothing when working with lye since lye can burn your skin.

Store your unused lye granules in a safe place because lye is a poison.

Remove your oil mixture from the heat and allow it to cool slightly to approximately 70 degrees.

You will probably want to customize the soap mixture with the ingredients that best meet your particular needs. The recipes on the following pages will give you some starter ideas. The ingredient list included in this books glossary will give you a much more comprehensive idea of which additives will work best for you.

While I do use additives that can prove beneficial for certain conditions, I typically do not add color or fragrance to any product designed for damaged or sensitive skin because additives can cause the irritation to worsen. If you prefer something other than the natural color or scent, you can add your favorite colorant, essential oils or herbs to the mixture.

Slowly pour the lye solution into the oil mixture. Stir until the ingredients are well blended

If the soap mixture does not thicken within 30 minutes or there is a greasy layer on the top of the mixture it may be too warm.

Set the container in a pan of cool Distilled Water. Stir the mixture, making certain that you stir the sides and bottom of the pan to ensure an even mix.

The mixture will become thicker taking on the consistency of syrup.

If the soap is lumpy, your mixture may be too cold. If this occurs, reverse the above process.

Sit the mixture in a pan of warm Distilled Water stirring until the lumps dissolve. Depending on the consistency you may need to replace your warm water more than once until the mixture is heated to the correct temperature for effective blending.

Pour the thickened mixture into your molds, cover, and keep the mixture in a warm place for at least 2 days. This helps keep the soap from separating.

Remember that everyone's skin reacts differently. You should test the products on a less sensitive area before using them. You should also remember that even natural products have side effects. The appendix gives the most common expected benefits and results of these ingredients. You should review these entries before trying any recipe.

Tallow Based Soaps

Tallow has been used for generations in soap making and is considered one of the most common homemade soap products. Tallow soaps are made using the fat by-product trimmed from meat. You can collect clean fat as you cook. Simply trim off clean beef or pork fat before you cook your meat and save it, preferably in the freezer, until you are ready to make soap. Your local butcher or meat department will often provide you with free fat that is left when they trim their products.

One bar of soap will need approximately 1 cup of clean fat. You can increase the recipe if you want to create a bigger batch.

Place the fat in your soap-making pan and heat it until it is melted to an oil form.

Allow your mixture to cool to approximately 115 degrees Fahrenheit.

Add 1 tsp. of borax powder for each cup of melted fat. You do not have to add borax but it does give a better appearance and lather to your soap. If you add the borax, stir the powder into your tallow mixture until well blended.

You will probably want to customize the soap mixture with the ingredients that best meet your particular needs. The recipes on the following pages will give you some starter ideas. The ingredient list included in this books glossary will give you a much more comprehensive idea of which additives will work best for you.

While I do use additives that can prove beneficial for certain conditions, I typically do not add color or fragrance to any product designed for damaged or sensitive skin because additives can cause the irritation to worsen. If you prefer something other than the natural color or scent, you can add your favorite colorant, essential oils or herbs to the mixture.

While your tallow mixture is cooling to the desired temperature, you will need to create the lye solution. Again, remember to wear protective gloves and clothing when using lye because it can burn the skin.

Lye is a poison and unused amounts should be stored in a safe place.

Dissolve the lye granules in cool Distilled Water.

You will use approximately 3 teaspoons of lye to ½ cup Distilled Water for each bar of soap being created.

Once the lye granules are dissolved, you will slowly pour the lye mixture into the fat mixture.

Pour it in a slow steady stream while stirring the mixture.

You should not have the heat on the mixture at this time.

Stir the ingredients until thick syrup is formed. This should take approximately 10-20 minutes.

If the soap is not becoming thick after 30 minutes or has a greasy layer floating on the top, the mixture may be too warm.

Set the container in a pan of cool Distilled Water.

Continue stirring, making sure to stir the sides and bottom of the pan to ensure an even mix.

If the soap is too lumpy, your mixture may be too cold.

If this occurs, reverse the above process.

Sit the mixture in a pan of warm Distilled Water stirring until the lumps dissolve.

Depending on the consistency of the mixture, you may need to replace your warm Distilled Water more than once until the soap is heated to the correct temperature.

Pour the thickened mixture into your molds, cover, and keep the mixture in a warm place for at least 2 days. This helps to keep the mixture from separating.

Once the soap has set, remove it from the molds and place it a dry area to age. Aging soap ensures a better quality final soap product. You should allow your tallow soap to age at least 2-3 weeks prior to use.

At times, you will find that your soap is lumpy or has separated during the aging process. If this occurs, do not throw out the failed soap.

Cut the flawed cakes of soap into small pieces. You can use an ordinary kitchen grater to cut the soap into smaller pieces.

Return the pieces to your soap-making pan and add approximately 1 cup of Distilled Water for each cake of ground soap.

Dissolve the soap in the Distilled Water over low heat. Stir the mixture occasionally to help distribute the heat.

When the lumps have disappeared and the mixture has formed a syrup, pour the soap into your favorite molds and follow the process for storage outlined earlier.

This will often cure the problem and provide you with a successful soap.

Remember that everyone's skin reacts differently. You should test the products on a less sensitive area before using them. You should also remember that even natural products have side effects. The appendix gives the most common expected benefits and results of these ingredients. You should review these entries before trying any recipe.

Glycerin Soap

One of the most common homemade cake soaps is a glycerin-based soap.

Glycerin is found naturally in many plants and is actually a by-product of the tallow soap making process. When making a fat and lye soap there is often a clear, thick liquid that floats on the top of the mixture. This is glycerin.

Glycerin soap is simply a basic soap that has extra glycerin added to the mixture. This soap is excellent for all skin types because it tends to be very mild. Glycerin is also natural humectant that draws and retains moisture in your skin.

The following recipe will make approximately 1 bar of soap. You can increase the recipe if you want to make a bigger batch.

Heat 1/3 cup of your favorite vegetable-based oil to approximately 80 degrees. Review the oil ingredient list to determine which oil will provide the most beneficial effect for your needs.

Add 1 tsp. of borax powder for each bar of soap you are making. You do not need to add the borax powder but it will make a nicer final product. If you choose to add the borax powder to your soap, stir the oils and borax until they are well blended.

While your oils are heating, dissolve 2 tsp. lye in 1/3 cup cold Distilled Water.

Remember to wear protective gloves and clothing when working with lye since it can burn your skin.

Store your unused lye granules in a safe place because lye is a poison.

Remove your oil mixture from the heat and allow it to cool to approximately 70 degrees.

You will probably want to customize the soap mixture with the ingredients that best meet your particular needs. The recipes on the following pages will give you some starter ideas. The ingredient list included in this books glossary will give you a much more comprehensive idea of which additives will work best for you.

While I do use additives that can prove beneficial for certain conditions, I typically do not add color or fragrance to any product designed for damaged or sensitive skin because additives can cause the irritation to worsen. If you prefer something other than the natural color or scent, you can add your favorite colorant, essential oils or herbs to the mixture.

Slowly pour the lye solution into the oil mixture.

Stir the mixture gently but mix well to ensure all of the ingredients are well blended.

When the ingredients are well blended, add 3 tsp. glycerin.

Continue stirring the mixture until the ingredients are well blended.

The mixture will take on the consistency of syrup.

If the soap mixture does not thicken within 30 minutes or if there is a greasy layer on the top of the mixture, it may be too warm.

Set the container in a pan of cool Distilled Water.

Continue stirring, making sure to stir the sides and bottom of the pan to ensure an even mix.

If the soap mixture is too lumpy, your mixture may be too cold. If this occurs, reverse the above process.

Sit the mixture in a pan of warm Distilled Water stirring until the lumps dissolve.

Depending on the consistency, you may need to replace your warm Distilled Water more than once until the lumps dissolve.

Pour the thickened mixture into your molds, cover, and keep it in a warm place for at least 2 days. This helps to keep the mixture from separating.

Remember that everyone's skin reacts differently. You should test the products on a less sensitive area before using them. You should also remember that even natural products have side effects. The appendix gives the most common expected benefits and results of these ingredients. You should review these entries before trying any recipe.

Soap Variations

The soap recipes on the following pages provide some customizations that you can use with the soap base recipes. You can create your own soap using the recipes on the previous pages, purchase melt-and-pour soap from a natural product supplier, or buy mass-market soap to use as a base. You will then customize these bases with ingredients that suit your particular skin care needs.

The variations on these pages are some of my favorite soap customizations. The ingredient mixes will work well with any of the core soap bases described earlier. At times, there is a soap base that works exceptionally well for a particular customization. These are noted in the recipe as a suggestion.

Remember that everyone's skin reacts differently. You should test the products on a less sensitive area before using them. You should also remember that even natural products have side effects. The appendix gives the most common expected benefits and results of these ingredients. You should review these entries before trying any recipe.

Do not be afraid to replace an ingredient in the customization recipes if you feel there is a better alternative for your needs. Creating your own natural products is all about experimentation and customization. You should strive to use the ingredients that meet your particular needs in every recipe.

Soothing Oatmeal Soap

Perhaps my favorite soap modification is to add oatmeal to make a soap that works to sooth my skin while giving a gentle exfoliation action. Oatmeal is gentle, soothing, and cleansing all at the same time. Oatmeal adds an exfoliating effect to the soap mixture while providing a soft, moist feel to the skin. This soap is perfect for removing oils & dead skin cells while soothing the irritation associated with acne. Liquid based oatmeal soap is very versatile so a Castile base is an excellent choice. I also love adding these ingredients to my coconut oil soap.

1 tsp.	Borax Powder
1/3 cup	Jojoba Oil
1 tsp.	Coconut Oil

Dissolve the borax powder in the oil base.

Borax in not a necessary ingredient for this recipe but it can improve the appearance and performance of your soap.

Heat the borax and oil mixture to approximately 80 degrees in your soap-making pan

Mix the ingredients well and add

3 tsp.	Glycerin
¼ cup	Ground Oatmeal
	Fragrance, Color, Emulsifier & Thickener as desired

While I do add herbs & oils that contain beneficial compounds, I typically do not add color or fragrance to any product designed for damaged skin because additives can cause the irritation to worsen. If you prefer something other than the natural color or scent, you can add your favorite colorant, essential oils or herbs to the mixture.

Pour the blended ingredients into your favorite soap base.

You may need to heat the mixture a second time before blending it with your soap base.

Continue stirring the mixture until the ingredients are well blended.

The mixture will become thicker as you stir. Pour the finished product into the soap molds of your choice and allow it to harden and age as directed by the soap base instructions.

Remember that everyone's skin reacts differently. You should test the products on a less sensitive area before using them. You should also remember that even natural products have side effects. The appendix gives the most common expected benefits and results of these ingredients. You should review these entries before trying any recipe.

Wake-up Bars

My husband loves this soap since he is a slow starter in the mornings. This soap has an invigorating smell that wakes him up. Better yet, this soap helps to tighten the skin, minimize the appearance of pores, and combat acne.

This recipe works well with liquid soap so Castile is often the preferred base but it works very well in any of the others. You can purchase ready-made castile soap and then customize the mixture to suit your needs or you may create castile soap at home. We like to create this recipe in liquid from and apply it with a scrubbing sack for the best benefits.

Create the soap base you have decided to use according to the recipe included earlier or buy pre-made soap from your favorite source. Add

2 tsp.   Camphor Oil

1 tsp   Mint Extract

While I do add herbs & oils that contain beneficial compounds, I typically do not add color or fragrance to any product designed for damaged skin because additives can cause the irritation to worsen. If you prefer something other than the natural color or scent, you can add your favorite colorant, essential oils or herbs to the mixture.

Stir the mixture well to ensure an even distribution of all of the ingredients.

If you are using this as a liquid application soap, shake the mixture well before each use.

If you are using a solid soap base, pour the finished product into the soap molds of your choice and allow it to harden and age as directed by the soap base instructions.

Remember that everyone's skin reacts differently. You should test the products on a less sensitive area before using them. You should also remember that even natural products have side effects. The appendix gives the most common expected benefits and results of these ingredients. You should review these entries before trying any recipe.

Oil Reducing Soap

This is one of the nicest soap customizations for treating clogged pores and extremely blemished skin. It helps to reduce excess oils while hydrating the skin to give it a beautiful glow. Many acne treatments dry the skin too much. This soap helps to infuse oils back into the skin. Jojoba oil is very similar to the natural oils produced by the body making it a nice moisturizer even for those who suffer from acne.

1/3 cup	Jojoba Oil
2 tbsp.	Baking Soda

Heat the jojoba oil to approximately 80 degrees. Add the baking soda and continue stirring until it dissolves in the oil.

Remove your oil mixture from the heat and allow it to cool to approximately 70 degrees.

Add the remaining ingredients and blend well.

3 tbsp.	Rose Water
3 tbsp.	Pineapple Juice
2 tbsp	Macadamia Nut Oil

While I do add herbs & oils that contain beneficial compounds, I typically do not add color or fragrance to any product designed for damaged skin because additives can cause the irritation to worsen. If you prefer something other than the natural color or scent, you can add your favorite colorant, essential oils or herbs to the mixture.

Pour the soap solution of your choice into the oil mixture and blend well.

The mixture will become thicker as you stir. Pour the finished product into the soap molds of your choice and allow it to harden and age as directed by the soap base instructions.

Remember that everyone's skin reacts differently. You should test the products on a less sensitive area before using them. You should also remember that even natural products have side effects. The appendix gives the most common expected benefits and results of these ingredients. You should review these entries before trying any recipe.

Super Skin Clearing Bars

This soap works especially well for those with acne caused by oily skin. I created this basic recipe for the teenagers in our family because it works very well at removing excess oils while clearing up skin blemishes caused by excess oil production.

1 tsp.	Borax Powder
2 tsp.	Sea Salt
3 tbsp.	Pineapple Juice
1 tbsp.	Honey

This modification works best with the beeswax soap base. You can select a different base to use if you wish. Heat the selected soap-base mixture as directed in the soap-making recipe.

Add the remaining ingredients, stirring until they are well blended

While I do add herbs & oils that contain beneficial compounds, I typically do not add color or fragrance to any product designed for damaged skin because additives can cause the irritation to worsen. If you prefer something other than the natural color or scent, you can add your favorite colorant, essential oils or herbs to the mixture.

The mixture will become thicker as you stir. Pour the finished product into the soap molds of your choice and allow it to harden and age as directed by the soap base instructions.

Remember that everyone's skin reacts differently. You should test the products on a less sensitive area before using them. You should also remember that even natural products have side effects. The appendix gives the most common expected benefits and results of these ingredients. You should review these entries before trying any recipe.

Clarifying Bars

I like to use this soap once a week year round to clarify and tighten my skin. It also adds a lovely glowing look while removing the impurities that can cause outbreaks. This recipe creates a bar soap as it is written. You can remove the beeswax from the instructions if you prefer a different soap base.

1/4 cup	Hazelnut Oil
2 tbsp.	Grated Beeswax
1 tbsp.	Honey

Heat the mixture to approximately 90 degrees.

Remove your base mixture from the heat and allow it to cool to approximately 70 degrees. Add

2 tbsp.	Orange Flower Distilled Water
2 tsp.	Baking Soda
1 tsp.	Aluminum Sulfate
1 tsp.	Borax Powder
2 tsp.	Grapefruit Juice

Use only *USP Grade for Cosmetic Use* Aluminum Sulfate products. Mix the ingredients in a plastic or ceramic dish using plastic utensils to avoid a reaction between the Aluminum Sulfate and the metal.

While I do add herbs & oils that contain beneficial compounds, I typically do not add color or fragrance to any product designed for damaged skin because additives can cause the irritation to worsen. If you prefer something other than the natural color or scent, you can add your favorite colorant, essential oils or herbs to the mixture.

Pour the soap solution of your choice into the oil mixture and blend well.

The mixture will become thicker as you stir. Pour the finished product into the soap molds of your choice and allow it to harden and age as directed by the soap base instructions.

Remember that everyone's skin reacts differently. You should test the products on a less sensitive area before using them. You should also remember that even natural products have side effects. The appendix gives the most common expected benefits and results of these ingredients. You should review these entries before trying any recipe.

Anti-Bacterial Bath Bars

Some types of acne can be caused or aggravated by bacteria. This is a wonderful alternative to some of the harsher anti-bacterial soaps on the market. These bath bars provide a gentle cleansing action while giving you additional skin protection against the bacterial and environmental irritants that often complicate acne outbreaks.

1/4 cup   Jojoba Oil

4 tsp.   Grated Beeswax

Place oils and beeswax in your soap-making pan and heat the mixture to approximately 90 degrees.

Remove your oil mixture from the heat and allow it to cool to approximately 70 degrees. Add

2 tbsp.   Honey

2 tbsp.   Glycerin

3 tbsp.   Lemon Juice

Stir the mixture until all of the ingredients are well blended.

While I do add herbs & oils that contain beneficial compounds, I typically do not add color or fragrance to any product designed for damaged skin because additives can cause the irritation to worsen. If you prefer something other than the natural color or scent, you can add your favorite colorant, essential oils or herbs to the mixture.

Pour the soap solution of your choice into the oil mixture and blend well.

The mixture will become thicker as you stir. Pour the finished product into the soap molds of your choice and allow it to harden and age as directed by the soap base instructions.

Remember that everyone's skin reacts differently. You should test the products on a less sensitive area before using them. You should also remember that even natural products have side effects. The appendix gives the most common expected benefits and results of these ingredients. You should review these entries before trying any recipe.

Bedtime Bars

This is a favorite of mine at night before bed. The natural aroma of lavender and chamomile provide a relaxing benefit, minimizing stress that might aggravate acne while the soap itself softens and hydrates the skin while killing bacteria and speeding the healing of blemishes. I typically follow this treatment with a hydrating moisturizer and wake with beautiful, moisturized skin. This soap modification works well with any of the soap base recipes but is written to use the beeswax base with a coconut oil foaming action. If you choose to use a different soap base, remove the beeswax and coconut oil from the following recipe.

1 tsp.	Chamomile Leaves
1 tsp.	Basil
1/4 cup	Distilled Water

Heat the Distilled Water to the boiling point and pour it over the leaves. Do not immerse the leaves in boiling Distilled Water since this might minimize the beneficial compounds contained in the plant parts. Allow the leaves and Distilled Water to soak overnight. The mixture should form a very strong tea. You can stain the plant parts from the mixture or leave them in to give added power to the finished soap.

1 tsp.	Borax Powder
3 tbsp.	Jojoba Oil
3 tsp.	Lavender Oil
3 tbsp.	Grated Beeswax
1 tbsp.	Coconut

Dissolve the borax powder in the oil base. Borax in not a necessary ingredient for this recipe but it can improve the appearance and performance of your soap.

Heat the borax and oil mixture to approximately 80 degrees in your soap-making pan.

Remove mixture from the heat and allow it to cool to approximately 70 degrees.

Blend the oils with the tea base. When the mixture is well blended, add the remaining ingredients.

1 tsp.   Lemon Juice

3 tsp.   Glycerin

While I do add herbs & oils that contain beneficial compounds, I typically do not add color or additional fragrance to any product designed for damaged skin because additives can cause the irritation to worsen. If you prefer something other than the natural color or scent, you can add your favorite colorant, essential oils or herbs to the mixture.

The mixture will become thicker as you stir. Pour the finished product into the soap molds of your choice and allow it to harden and age as directed by the soap base instructions.

Remember that everyone's skin reacts differently. You should test the products on a less sensitive area before using them. You should also remember that even natural products have side effects. The appendix gives the most common expected benefits and results of these ingredients. You should review these entries before trying any recipe.

Hydrating Apple Soap

Hydration is essential for beautiful, healthy skin and this soap not only infuses the skin with moisture it also helps to sooth irritation. This is a great choice when you have itchy, irritated acne outbreaks. This modification works very well with a beeswax soap base. The juice helps to attract moisture, the beeswax protects from irritants, and the chlorophyll speeds healing.

Create the soap base of your choice according to the instructions. Add

2 tbsp.   Apple Juice

1 tsp.   Liquid Chlorophyll

The mixture will have a delicate apple scent and a lovely green color. If you desire a different color or fragrance, you may add food coloring or the desired essential oils to the mixture.

While I do add herbs & oils that contain beneficial compounds, I typically do not add color or fragrance to any product designed for damaged skin because additives can cause the irritation to worsen.

The mixture will become thicker as you stir. Pour the finished product into the soap molds of your choice and allow it to harden and age as directed by the soap base instructions.

Remember that everyone's skin reacts differently. You should test the products on a less sensitive area before using them. You should also remember that even natural products have side effects. The appendix gives the most common expected benefits and results of these ingredients. You should review these entries before trying any recipe.

Exfoliating Bars

This soap is an excellent choice when you want a soap that will hydrate and exfoliate all in one. It helps to remove dead skin cells, oils, and dirt while leaving the skin looking and feeling clean & refreshed. You will be amazed at how moist and clear you skin looks after using this soap.

1 tsp.	Borax Powder
1/3 cup	Hazelnut Oil
1 tsp.	Coconut Oil
2 tsp.	Grated Beeswax

Melt the beeswax until it reaches around 90 degrees Fahrenheit and has a liquid appearance. Remove the beeswax from the heat and add the borax powder & oil to the base. Borax in not a necessary ingredient for this recipe but it can improve the appearance and performance of your soap.

Add

2 tsp.	Lye Granules
1/3 cup	Cold Distilled Water
1/8 cup	Carrot Juice

Stir the mixture until the ingredients are well blended.

The mixture will have an orange appearance. If you desire a specific color or fragrance for your soap, you may add your favorite food coloring or essential oils.

While I do add herbs & oils that contain beneficial compounds, I typically do not add color or fragrance to any product designed for damaged skin because additives can cause the irritation to worsen.

Pour the soap solution of your choice into the base. You can simply increase the amount of beeswax too instead of adding a soap base. This will help the mixture to solidify.

When the ingredients are well blended, add the remaining ingredients.

3 tsp.   Glycerin

1   Orange Peel grated medium fine

Continue stirring the mixture until well blended. The mixture will become thicker taking on the consistency of syrup.

The mixture will become thicker as you stir. Pour the finished product into the soap molds of your choice and allow it to harden and age as directed by the soap base instructions.

Remember that everyone's skin reacts differently. You should test the products on a less sensitive area before using them. You should also remember that even natural products have side effects. The appendix gives the most common expected benefits and results of these ingredients. You should review these entries before trying any recipe.

Scar Reduction Bars

Once you have an outbreak under control, the dark pigmentation left behind can really affect your appearance. This soap helps to treat the outbreaks while fading dark pigmentation scarring.

1/4 cup	Jojoba Oil
2 tbsp.	Grated Beeswax
1 tbsp.	Honey

Heat the mixture to approximately 90 degrees until it reaches a syrupy consistency.

Remove your oil mixture from the heat and allow it to cool to approximately 70 degrees.   Add

2 tbsp.	Bitter Damson - Powdered
½ tsp.	Lilac Oil
½ tsp.	Patchouli Oil

While I do add herbs & oils that contain beneficial compounds, I typically do not add color or fragrance to any product designed for damaged skin because additives can cause the irritation to worsen. If you prefer something other than the natural color or scent, you can add your favorite colorant, essential oils or herbs to the mixture.

Pour the soap solution of your choice into the oil mixture and blend well.

The mixture will become thicker as you stir. Pour the finished product into the soap molds of your choice and allow it to harden and age as directed by the soap base instructions.

Remember that everyone's skin reacts differently. You should test the products on a less sensitive area before using them. You should also remember that even natural products have side effects. The appendix gives the most common expected benefits and results of these ingredients. You should review these entries before trying any recipe.

Moisture Infusing Bars

This is a fantastic cleanser for either waterless use throughout the day or incorporated into a soap base like glycerin. The recipe provides a mild anti-bacterial effect while giving your skin the moisture & protection it needs to heal.

4 tbsp   Rose Water

2 tbsp   Glycerin

Heat the rose water and glycerin in a microwave safe dish for 45 seconds or use a double boiler to bring the mixture to approximately 90 degrees Fahrenheit.

¼ tsp   Borax Powder

Dissolve borax into heated liquid. Stir gently to prevent foaming.

¼ cup   Aloe Vera Gel

Slowly pour the mixture into an aloe base and stir until all ingredients are well blended.

While I do add herbs & oils that contain beneficial compounds, I typically do not add color or fragrance to any product designed for damaged skin because additives can cause the irritation to worsen. If you prefer something other than the natural color or scent, you can add your favorite colorant, essential oils or herbs to the mixture.

Pour the finished solution into your slightly cooled soap base and blend well.

The mixture will become thicker as you stir. Pour the finished product into the soap molds of your choice and allow it to harden and age as directed by the soap base instructions.

If you want to try this as a quick, Distilled Waterless application, you can leave out the soap base and pour the finished mixture into your favorite applicator container – this mixture also pumps well.

Remember that everyone's skin reacts differently. You should test the products on a less sensitive area before using them. You should also remember that even natural products have side effects. The appendix gives the most common expected benefits and results of these ingredients. You should review these entries before trying any recipe.

Soft Soaps & Cleansers

Every inch of your skin is important and deserves to be treated with care but areas that are acne prone require specialized attention. Soft soaps and cleansers are a preferred choice for some people, especially when treating facial acne. Soft cleansers help to remove the dirt, oils, bacteria, and other toxins that contribute to acne outbreaks without further aggravating the already sensitive skin.

Cleansing is one of the best places that you can spend time experimenting and customizing the recipes to suit your needs. The better customized your cleansing regimen is to your particular skin type, lifestyle, and needs the better your overall appearance will be.

You may need to use different cleansers on different parts of your skin. Facial acne tends to be a slightly different problem than back acne and will need different treatments and preventatives. You should consider the underlying cause of the acne, sensitivity of the areas being treated, and personal application preferences before selecting recipes to try.

Regardless of the recipes you choose to try it is always recommended that you test sample the products on a sensitive area such as your wrist to ensure that you do not have unexpected reactions before applying them to your skin. This is not a fail proof method of ensuring that the products are correct for you but it can often provide a warning of a negative reaction.

You should also look up each ingredient in the ingredient listing to determine potential side effects of using any natural product. Natural products contain medicinal qualities and you need to ensure that each inclusion is safe and effective for your personal needs.

Foaming Daily Scrub

Foaming washes are one of my favorite types of facial cleansers. The foaming action helps to clean the skin and makes application a breeze. This is a favorite cleaner of mine since it is gentle enough for year round use and the natural ingredients help to tighten my skin, combat the severity of outbreaks, and improve the overall look and texture of my skin.

3 tbsp.   Birch Bark Tea

3 tbsp.   Witch Hazel

Blend the ingredients in a blender or food processor until they are smooth. Add

1 tbsp.   Coconut Oil

               Emulsifier & Thickener as desired

Gently stir the coconut oil into the mixture until all of the ingredients are well blended.

Do not whip this mixture since the coconut oil will foam.

This recipe has a delicate, sweet smell but if you desire a specific color or fragrance, you may add your favorite colorant or essential oils or herbs to the mixture.

While I do add herbs & oils that contain beneficial compounds, I typically do not add color or fragrance to any product designed for damaged skin because additives can cause the irritation to worsen.

Spoon mixture into a clean container and seal it tightly.

To use, place a small amount in the palm of your hand, mix with Distilled Water, and scrub your face with a gentle upward motion.

Remember that everyone's skin reacts differently. You should test the products on a less sensitive area before using them. You should also remember that even natural products have side effects. The appendix gives the most common expected benefits and results of these ingredients. You should review these entries before trying any recipe.

Dermabrasion Scrub

This mildly abrasive cleanser helps to remove surface dirt, oils, and dead skin cells while helping to reduce the bacteria that may be a factor in acne. Oatmeal is a good component selection since it provides a gentle cleansing action without the harsh effects of some other abrasives. This recipe includes my favorite ingredients but you might want to refer to the appendix for ingredient ideas that will work better with your personal acne needs.

1 cup	Warm Distilled Water
1 tsp	Black Thorn Flowers

Bring the Distilled Water to a light boil.

Remove the Distilled Water from the heat.

Add the blackthorn flowers.

Allow the mixture to steep for 4-6 hours creating a strong infusion.

Strain the flowers from the mixture. Discard the flowers but keep the liquid as the base for your cleanser.

½ cup	Uncooked Oatmeal
½ tsp	Bayberry Oil
1 tbsp	Glycerin
2 drops	Tincture of Benzoin
	Emulsifier & Thickener as desired

Place all of the ingredients in a blender or food processor.

Mix the ingredients for approximately 2 minutes or until a pasty texture has been achieved.

While I do add herbs & oils that contain beneficial compounds, I typically do not add color or fragrance to any product designed for damaged skin because additives can cause the irritation to worsen. If you prefer something other than the natural color or scent, you can add your favorite colorant, essential oils or herbs to the mixture.

Store the finished mixture in a tightly sealed container

To apply, place a small amount into the palm of your hand and massage it into the face and skin in an upward motion.

Rinse your skin well and pat dry.

This gentle cleanser works well for all skin types. This mixture may be used on the face and body.

Remember that everyone's skin reacts differently. You should test the products on a less sensitive area before using them. You should also remember that even natural products have side effects. The appendix gives the most common expected benefits and results of these ingredients. You should review these entries before trying any recipe.

Daily Clarifying Cleanser

If your skin is naturally dry, you may not need much in the way of clarifying washes or rinses. Most acne sufferers do get an oily build-up. If this is the case with your skin, you will want to add a clarifying wash every couple of days to help alleviate dullness and remove some of the excess oils, toxins and dried skin that can contribute to the severity of an outbreak.

½ cup	Aloe Vera Gel
1 tbsp.	Black Seed Oil
1 tbsp.	Caje Oil
3 tbsp.	Witch Hazel
¼ tsp.	Tincture of Benzoin
	Emulsifier & Thickener as desired

Mix the ingredients in a blender or food processor until they are well blended.

While I do add herbs & oils that contain beneficial compounds, I typically do not add color or fragrance to any product designed for damaged skin because additives can cause the irritation to worsen. If you prefer something other than the natural color or scent, you can add your favorite colorant, essential oils or herbs to the mixture.

Store the mixture in a tightly sealed container

To use, massage a small amount into your skin using an upward motion.

Let the mixture sit on the skin for 30 – 60 seconds before rinsing.

Remember that everyone's skin reacts differently. You should test the products on a less sensitive area before using them. You should also remember that even natural products have side effects. The appendix gives the most common expected benefits and results of these ingredients. You should review these entries before trying any recipe.

Daily Cleanser with Toning Agents

This recipe visibly reduces the appearance of pores while helping to combat the severity of an acne outbreak. It also helps to heal damaged skin while giving a light toning action. I modify the recipe by adding ingredients from the alternate ingredient list throughout the year to get the most beneficial results for each season. You can use this cleanser alone or add additional ingredients from the list to ensure the best results for your skin type.

2 tbsp.	Carob Powder
3 tsp.	Honey
¼ cup	Witch Hazel
1 tsp .	Borax Powder
1 tbsp.	Atlas Cedar Oil
	Emulsifier & Thickener as desired

Mix the ingredients in a food processor or stir by hand until they are well blended.

While I do add herbs & oils that contain beneficial compounds, I typically do not add color or fragrance to any product designed for damaged skin because additives can cause the irritation to worsen. If you prefer something other than the natural color or scent, you can add your favorite colorant, essential oils or herbs to the mixture.

Store the finished mixture in a tightly sealed container. A pump bottles work well with this base. To use, pump a pea sized drop into the palm of your hand and massage it into your skin using an upward motion. Allow the cleanser to sit on your skin for 30-60 seconds before rinsing.

Remember that everyone's skin reacts differently. You should test the products on a less sensitive area before using them. You should also remember that even natural products have side effects. The appendix gives the most common expected benefits and results of these ingredients. You should review these entries before trying any recipe.

Daily Moisturizing Antibacterial Cleanser

This light cleanser combines a mild anti-bacterial effect with a very gentle cleansing action. It makes a good selection for preventative daily cleansing.

½ cup	Castile Soap
1/8 cup	Honey
1 tbsp	Fresh Lemon Juice
3 drops	Tincture of Benzoin

Mix all of the ingredients until they are well blended.

While I do add herbs & oils that contain beneficial compounds, I typically do not add color or fragrance to any product designed for damaged skin because additives can cause the irritation to worsen. If you prefer something other than the natural color or scent, you can add your favorite colorant, essential oils or herbs to the mixture.

Pour the finished mixture into your favorite applicator bottle.

This is a soap mixture so always rinse your skin thoroughly when done washing.

Castile soap can be made at home following the basic recipe in the soap making section.

Remember that everyone's skin reacts differently. You should test the products on a less sensitive area before using them. You should also remember that even natural products have side effects. The appendix gives the most common expected benefits and results of these ingredients. You should review these entries before trying any recipe.

Lavender Moisturizing Antibacterial Wash

This is a fantastic nighttime cleanser. Lavender gives a soothing effect helping to combat stress reactions that may be a contributing factor in an acne outbreak. It also helps to inhibit bacterial growth that can sometimes complicate acne. The other ingredients tighten, tone, and heal the skin. I also use this cleanser as a bath additive when I need a relaxing bath to help prepare for bed or a full body cleanser.

¼ tsp	Tincture of Benzoin
1 tbsp	Distilled Water
3 tbsp	Witch Hazel
3-4 drops	Lavender Oil
1 tsp	Glycerin
3 tbsp	Aloe Vera Gel

Gently combine all of the ingredients until they well blended.

This mixture will have an interesting scent resulting from the blend of lavender, witch hazel and aloe. If you want something more than the natural scent & color, you can add your preferred herb, oil, or colorant now.

While I do add herbs & oils that contain beneficial compounds, I typically do not add color or fragrance to any product designed for damaged skin because additives can cause the irritation to worsen.

Pour the finished mixture into your favorite dispenser container. A pump dispenser works well with this mixture. To use, pump a pea sized amount of cleanser into the palm of your hand and massage into your skin using a gentle upward motion. Allow the cleanser to sit on your skin 30-60 seconds before rinsing.

Remember that everyone's skin reacts differently. You should test the products on a less sensitive area before using them. You should also remember that even natural products have side effects. The appendix gives the most common expected benefits and results of these ingredients. You should review these entries before trying any recipe.

Foaming Anti-bacterial Scrub

This foaming wash combines a gentle cleansing agent with anti-bacterial benefits and easy application. It is my first choice for a quick cleanser especially when I am trying to combat enlarged pores.

3 tbsp	Coconut Oil
1 tsp	Grapefruit Juice
1 tsp	Honey
3 tbsp	Witch Hazel
¼ tsp	Tincture of Benzoin
1 crushed	Vitamin C Tablet

Dissolve the Vitamin C powder in the witch hazel mixture.

Add the remaining ingredients and stir gently until they are well blended.

The mixture will foam if it is stirred too vigorously.

While I do add herbs & oils that contain beneficial compounds, I typically do not add color or fragrance to any product designed for damaged skin because additives can cause the irritation to worsen. If you prefer something other than the natural color or scent, you can add your favorite colorant, essential oils or herbs to the mixture.

Pour the finished mixture into a tightly sealed container. To use, apply a small amount of the cleanser to your skin using a gentle upward motion. Rinse well and pat the skin dry.

Remember that everyone's skin reacts differently. You should test the products on a less sensitive area before using them. You should also remember that even natural products have side effects. The appendix gives the most common expected benefits and results of these ingredients. You should review these entries before trying any recipe.

Soothing Cleansing Balm

This cleanser acts as a gentle, moisturizing balm that soothes and protects your skin. It is especially useful for people who suffer from seborrhea or as a balm when other treatments have dried out the skin.

¼ cup	Aloe Vera Gel
1 tbsp.	Vitamin E Oil
2 tbsp.	Borax Powder
2 tbsp.	Powdered Milk
¼ cup	Witch Hazel

Dissolve borax and milk powders in the witch hazel base. Add the remaining ingredients and blend well.

While I do add herbs & oils that contain beneficial compounds, I typically do not add color or fragrance to any product designed for damaged skin because additives can cause the irritation to worsen. If you prefer something other than the natural color or scent, you can add your favorite colorant, essential oils or herbs to the mixture.

Pour the finished mixture into clean container and seal tightly.

To use, pour small amount in the palm of your hand or apply it with a gentle upward motion. Allow the mixture to sit on your skin for 30-60 seconds before rinsing. This is also an excellent cleanser to add to your favorite scrubbing sacks.

Remember that everyone's skin reacts differently. You should test the products on a less sensitive area before using them. You should also remember that even natural products have side effects. The appendix gives the most common expected benefits and results of these ingredients. You should review these entries before trying any recipe.

Soothing Wash

This is one of the more soothing skin washes. It works best when acne outbreaks are most severe. It helps to hydrate while easing the inflammation of an outbreak.

1 tbsp.   Marshmallow Root

1 cup   Distilled Water

Marshmallow Root tends to respond best as a cold infusion. The Distilled Water should be warm, not hot when you add the root. Place the mixture in a cool place and allow the root to steep for up to 24 hours. Strain the marshmallow root from the liquid and discard the plant parts. The liquid will act as a base for your cleanser.

3 tsp.   Aloe Vera Gel

1 tsp.   Cedarwood Oil

1 tsp.   Geranium Oil

                Emulsifier & Thickener as desired

Add the remaining ingredients to the marshmallow root fluid and stir the mixture until it is well blended.

While I do add herbs & oils that contain beneficial compounds, I typically do not add color or fragrance to any product designed for damaged skin because additives can cause the irritation to worsen. If you prefer something other than the natural color or scent, you can add your favorite colorant, essential oils, or herbs to the mixture.

Pour the finished cleanser into a clean, dry bottle with a tight fitting lid

The mixture will separate if it is left standing so shake the cleanser well before each use.

Apply the cleanser to the skin with a cotton ball as an astringent wash up to 3 times daily. You do not need to rinse this cleanser completely from the skin.

Remember that everyone's skin reacts differently. You should test the products on a less sensitive area before using them. You should also remember that even natural products have side effects. The appendix gives the most common expected benefits and results of these ingredients. You should review these entries before trying any recipe.

Healing Cleanser

This is an excellent cleansing gel for both the face and the body. We use it whenever our skin is overstressed, irritated, or we just need a bit of skin help. The arrowroot powder helps to condition the skin aiding it in retaining moisture while promoting healing. The glycerin attracts moisture, promoting repair of the damage and helps to give a hydrated, supple look to the skin.

2 tbsp.	Abscess Root
2 cups	Distilled Water
1 tbsp.	Apple Cider Vinegar
2 tbsp.	Glycerin
	Emulsifier & Thickener as desired

Heat the Distilled Water to a boil. Remove the Distilled Water from the heat and add the Abscess Root. Allow the mixture to steep for 4 – 6 hours until a dark infusion has been made. You can strain the abscess root from the mixture or leave it in to obtain the most benefit from the compounds.

Mix the vinegar & glycerin into the solution, stirring gently until all of the ingredients are well blended.

While I do add herbs & oils that contain beneficial compounds, I typically do not add color or fragrance to any product designed for damaged skin because additives can cause the irritation to worsen. If you prefer something other than the natural color or scent, you can add your favorite colorant, essential oils or herbs to the mixture.

Store the finished cleanser in a tightly sealed container, preferably in the refrigerator. To use, apply a small amount to your skin using a gentle upward motion. Allow the mixture to soak into the skin for 30-60 seconds before rinsing.

Remember that everyone's skin reacts differently. You should test the products on a less sensitive area before using them. You should also remember that even natural products have side effects. The appendix gives the most common expected benefits and results of these ingredients. You should review these entries before trying any recipe.

Inflammation Wash

This wash helps to sooth inflammation and irritation while combating the most common causes of acne outbreaks.

1 tbsp.	Powdered Agrimony
1 cup	Distilled Water
3 tsp.	Aloe Vera Gel
1 tsp.	Arnica Tincture
1 tsp.	Geranium Oil
	Emulsifier & Thickener as desired

Mix the ingredients using a blender or whisk.

While I do add herbs & oils that contain beneficial compounds, I typically do not add color or fragrance to any product designed for damaged skin because additives can cause the irritation to worsen. If you prefer something other than the natural color or scent, you can add your favorite colorant, essential oils, or herbs to the mixture.

Pour the mixture into a clean, dry bottle with a tight fitting lid

The mixture will separate if it is left standing so shake the cleanser well before each use.

Apply to skin with a cotton ball as an astringent wash up to 3 times daily.

Remember that everyone's skin reacts differently. You should test the products on a less sensitive area before using them. You should also remember that even natural products have side effects. The appendix gives the most common expected benefits and results of these ingredients. You should review these entries before trying any recipe.

Extreme Wash with Healing Properties

This recipe makes one of the most drying washes of any of the recipes. It helps to reduce seepage associated with certain types of acne outbreaks. You should use caution with this wash since it can have an excessive drying effect. It does have properties that help to stimulate healing so if your skin is extremely oily with active outbreaks, this may be the most effective relief wash for your particular needs.

½ cup	Rose Water
¼ cup	Witch Hazel
1 tsp.	Aloe Vera Gel
1 tsp.	Liquid Chlorophyll
1 tsp.	Grapefruit Seed Oil
	Emulsifier & Thickener as desired

While I do add herbs & oils that contain beneficial compounds, I typically do not add color or fragrance to any product designed for damaged skin because additives can cause the irritation to worsen. If you prefer something other than the natural color or scent, you can add your favorite colorant, essential oils, or herbs to the mixture.

Pour the mixture into a clean, dry bottle with a tight fitting lid

The mixture will separate if it is left standing so shake the cleanser well before each use.

Apply to skin with a cotton ball as an astringent wash up to 3 times daily.

Remember that everyone's skin reacts differently. You should test the products on a less sensitive area before using them. You should also remember that even natural products have side effects. The appendix gives the most common expected benefits and results of these ingredients. You should review these entries before trying any recipe.

Seborrhea & Acne Cleanser

This cleanser works well at combating acne complicated by seborrhea. The yogurt infuses moisture into the skin while the lemon juice & sweet gale oils help to restore the skins natural acid levels minimizing acne outbreaks and brightening the complexion.

½ cup	Unflavored Yogurt
1 tbsp	Sweet Gale Oil
2 tsp	Lemon Juice
	Emulsifier & Thickener as desired

Whip all of the ingredients in a blender or by hand until they are well blended.

While I do add herbs & oils that contain beneficial compounds, I typically do not add color or fragrance to any product designed for damaged skin because additives can cause the irritation to worsen. If you prefer something other than the natural color or scent, you can add your favorite colorant, essential oils or herbs to the mixture.

Pour a small amount in the palm of your hand, massage gently into the skin using an upward motion. This cleanser should be allowed to set into the skin for at least 1 minute before rinsing.

Store the extra cleanser in the refrigerator since the yogurt will spoil.

Remember that everyone's skin reacts differently. You should test the products on a less sensitive area before using them. You should also remember that even natural products have side effects. The appendix gives the most common expected benefits and results of these ingredients. You should review these entries before trying any recipe.

Cleansing Soap for Seborrhea

This great moisturizing cleanser helps to reduce the severity of seborrhea without adding irritants that may aggravate the skin. It also works exceptionally well at restoring tone and moisture to overstressed skin.

1 tsp.	Borax Powder
3 tbsp.	Distilled Water
½ tsp.	Damask Rose
½ tsp.	Sweet Gale
¼ cup	Aloe Vera Gel
	Emulsifier & Thickener as desired

Dissolve the borax powder in the Distilled Water.

Mix the borax Distilled Water with the remaining ingredients until a creamy gel has formed.

While I do add herbs & oils that contain beneficial compounds, I typically do not add color or fragrance to any product designed for damaged skin because additives can cause the irritation to worsen. If you prefer something other than the natural color or scent, you can add your favorite colorant, essential oils or herbs to the mixture.

Store the mixture in a tightly sealed container.

Remember that everyone's skin reacts differently. You should test the products on a less sensitive area before using them. You should also remember that even natural products have side effects. The appendix gives the most common expected benefits and results of these ingredients. You should review these entries before trying any recipe.

Anti-Septic Cleansing Gel

This wonderful gel helps to combat bacteria and minimizes future outbreaks while speeding healing of your current outbreak.

2 tbsp.	Acacia Bark Powder
2 tsp.	Powdered Burdock Leaves
¼ cup	Distilled Water
¼ cup	Aloe Vera Gel
2 tbsp.	Glycerin
	Emulsifier & Thickener as desired

Dissolve the powders in the Distilled Water. You may need to heat the powder and Distilled Water mixture to help with the blending process. I like to use a double boiler for this process since I can continuously stir the mixture while the powders dissolve. The liquid will thicken slightly as you stir it.

If the mixture becomes thicker than you want, you may add additional Distilled Water until you obtain the consistency you prefer.

Mix the glycerin & aloe vera into the solution stirring gently until all of the ingredients are well blended.

While I do add herbs & oils that contain beneficial compounds, I typically do not add color or fragrance to any product designed for damaged skin because additives can cause the irritation to worsen. If you prefer something other than the natural color or scent, you can add your favorite colorant, essential oils or herbs to the mixture.

Remember that everyone's skin reacts differently. You should test the products on a less sensitive area before using them. You should also remember that even natural products have side effects. The appendix gives the most common expected benefits and results of these ingredients. You should review these entries before trying any recipe.

Basic Daily Cleanser

This cleanser is mildly astringent with the juices helping to clarify oily skin. The honey acts to repair damage and combat bacterial. The ingredients also aid in the prevention of future outbreaks.

1 tsp.	Borax powder
¼ cup	Distilled Water

Heat the borax and water in a microwave safe dish until they are just boiling. Add

2 tbsp.	Grapefruit juice
2 tsp.	Camphor
1 tsp.	Carrot Oil
1 tsp.	Geranium
	Emulsifier & Thickener as desired

Stir the mixture until all of the ingredients are well blended.

This mixture will be slightly looser than the other cleansers so you may wish to add a thickening agent for easier application.

This recipe has a lovely sweet smell and a pretty color but if you desire a specific color or fragrance, you may add your favorite colorant or essential oils or herbs to the mixture.

While I do add herbs & oils that contain beneficial compounds, I typically do not add color or fragrance to any product designed for damaged skin because additives can cause the irritation to worsen.

Pour the mixture into a clean container and seal tightly. To apply, pour a small amount into the palm of your hand and gently massage into the face with upward motions. Rinse the skin and pat dry.

Remember that everyone's skin reacts differently. You should test the products on a less sensitive area before using them. You should also remember that even natural products have side effects. The appendix gives the most common expected benefits and results of these ingredients. You should review these entries before trying any recipe.

Beauty Milk Cleanser

Milk has been used as a beauty treatment for thousands of years. This milk cleanser is excellent for infusing the skin with moisture while aiding in the restoration of the skin's natural PH. The wash helps to minimize the likelihood of outbreaks while improving both the texture and appearance of the skin.

¼ cup	Dry Milk Powder
2 tbsp.	Rose Water
2 tbsp.	Cajuput Oil
2 tsp.	Lemon Juice
	Emulsifier & Thickener as desired

Place all of the ingredients in a blender and mix until a thick paste is formed.

If the finished mixture is too thick, you may add a few extra drops of Distilled Water until the desired consistency is obtained.

While I do add herbs & oils that contain beneficial compounds, I typically do not add color or fragrance to any product designed for damaged skin because additives can cause the irritation to worsen. If you prefer something other than the natural color or scent, you can add your favorite colorant, essential oils, or herbs to the mixture.

The resulting mixture will be a thick paste. Spoon the mixture into a clean container and seal it tightly. Refrigeration may lengthen the shelf life of the product.

To use, place a small amount of the paste in the palm of your hand and add additional water as needed. Apply the resulting mixture in an upward motion into your skin. Allow the cleanser to sit on the skin for 30-60 seconds before rinsing.

Remember that everyone's skin reacts differently. You should test the products on a less sensitive area before using them. You should also remember that even natural products have side effects. The appendix gives the most common expected benefits and results of these ingredients. You should review these entries before trying any recipe.

Sweet Radiance Cleanser

Acne prone skin can still have a well-hydrated, radiant glow. I love to use this one whenever I need a refreshed look. Most people who suffer from acne forget that hydration is sometimes as important to the health of your skin as acne specific treatments.

2 tbsp.	Plain Yogurt
1 tsp.	Honey
1 tbsp.	Geranium Oil
1 tbsp.	Fennel Oil
1 tbsp.	Rose Water (you may use Witch Hazel if desired)
	Emulsifier & Thickener as desired

Place all of the ingredients in a blender and mix until a thick paste is formed.

If the finished mixture is too thick, you may add a few drops of distilled water or a bit more rosewater until the desired consistency is obtained.

While I do add herbs & oils that contain beneficial compounds, I typically do not add color or fragrance to any product designed for damaged skin because additives can cause the irritation to worsen. This cleanser has a beautiful, light fragrance of its own, but if you desire a specific color or fragrance, you may add your favorite colorant or essential oils or herbs to the mixture

Spoon the mixture into a clean container and seal it tightly.

Refrigeration may lengthen the shelf life of the product. This recipe makes one or two applications. If you choose to enlarge the recipe, refrigeration is necessary.

To use, place a small amount of the paste in the palm of your hand and apply to your skin in an upward motion. Allow the cleanser to sit on the 30-60 seconds before rinsing.

Remember that everyone's skin reacts differently. You should test the products on a less sensitive area before using them. You should also remember that even natural products have side effects. The appendix gives the most common expected benefits and results of these ingredients. You should review these entries before trying any recipe.

Skin Smoothing Cleanser

This is an excellent cleaner that I like to use in the winter months when my skin can begin to look dull and blotchy or if it suffers from what we call winter acne. It helps to tighten and tone my skin while improving the texture. It also acts to combat acne outbreaks and speed healing of current outbreaks.

½ cup	Aloe Vera Gel
1 tbsp.	Powdered Milk
¼ cup	Witch Hazel
2 tbsp.	Camphor Oil
1 tbsp.	Jojoba Oil
	Emulsifier & Thickener as desired

Mix all of the ingredients in a blender until a gel has formed.

The mixture will be looser and works very well in a pump. You may want to consider adding a beneficial thickening agent like Acacia Powder to the mixture for easier application.

While I do add herbs & oils that contain beneficial compounds, I typically do not add color or fragrance to any product designed for damaged skin because additives can cause the irritation to worsen. If you prefer something other than the natural color or scent, you can add your favorite colorant, essential oils, or herbs to the mixture.

To use apply a small amount to your skin massaging in an upward motion. Allow the cleanser to sit on the skin for 30-60 seconds before rinsing.

Remember that everyone's skin reacts differently. You should test the products on a less sensitive area before using them. You should also remember that even natural products have side effects. The appendix gives the most common expected benefits and results of these ingredients. You should review these entries before trying any recipe.

Acne Control & Scar Reduction Wash

This wash acts as both a treatment & preventive against eruptions while helping to fade the scarring associated with healed outbreaks.

1 tsp	Burdock Root
1/2 cup	Distilled Water

Bring the Distilled Water to a boil and remove it from the heat. Add the burdock root and allow the mixture to steep for 4-6 hours. You can strain the plant parts from the liquid or leave them in to make a more powerful cleanser. Add:

½ cup	Witch Hazel
2 tsp	Aloe Vera Gel
2 tsp	Calendula Oil
1 tsp	Cedarwood Oil
	Emulsifier & Thickener as desired

While I do add herbs & oils that contain beneficial compounds, I typically do not add color or fragrance to any product designed for damaged skin because additives can cause the irritation to worsen. If you prefer something other than the natural color or scent, you can add your favorite colorant, essential oils, or herbs to the mixture.

Pour the mixture into a clean, dry bottle with a tight fitting lid.

The mixture will separate if it is left standing so shake the cleanser well before each use.

Apply to the skin with a cotton ball as an astringent wash up to 3 times daily.

Remember that everyone's skin reacts differently. You should test the products on a less sensitive area before using them. You should also remember that even natural products have side effects. The appendix gives the most common expected benefits and results of these ingredients. You should review these entries before trying any recipe.

Scar Reduction Cleanser

Sometimes, the dark pigmentation left behind after an outbreak can be as much of a problem as the acne itself. This wonderful, soothing cleanser helps to reduce the appearance of dark pigmentation scars with the added bonus of working to prevent future outbreaks.

½ cup	Aloe Vera Gel
½ cup	Milk of Papaya
½ tsp.	Rose Hip Oil
3 tbsp.	Witch Hazel
¼ tsp.	Tincture of Benzoin
	Emulsifier & Thickener as desired

Mix the ingredients in a blender or food processor until they are well blended.

While I do add herbs & oils that contain beneficial compounds, I typically do not add color or fragrance to any product designed for damaged skin because additives can cause the irritation to worsen. If you prefer something other than the natural color or scent, you can add your favorite colorant, essential oils, or herbs to the mixture.

Store the finished cleanser in a tightly sealed container, preferably in the refrigerator.

To use massage a small amount into your skin using an upward motion. Allow the cleanser to sit on the skin 30 – 60 seconds before rinsing.

Remember that everyone's skin reacts differently. You should test the products on a less sensitive area before using them. You should also remember that even natural products have side effects. The appendix gives the most common expected benefits and results of these ingredients. You should review these entries before trying any recipe.

CHAPTER 3

Exfoliating Scrubs

Sometimes dirt, oils, and dead skin cells build up on the skin. An exfoliating cleanser helps remove the build up and condition the skin in preparation for other treatments. Exfoliation is the act of lightly abrading the skin to help remove dead skin cells and reveal new, healthy skin cells.

Exfoliation is an important step toward obtaining the healthy, glowing skin you desire. Exfoliation not only removes dead cells and impurities, but the process of removing these cells actually allows your skin to retain moisture.

These specialized products may be used in place of or in addition to your regular cleanser.

Abrasive cleansers can irritate some types of acne and seborrhea so you should use caution the first time you try an exfoliating cleanser. Other outbreaks can actually be the result of a build up of dead skin cells & oils and an exfoliating cleanser is needed to begin the treatment process. You should always test any new product before using it to determine exactly how your skin will react. If your test patch tolerates the scrub well, try using it a few times a week and see how much better your daily treatments perform.

Remember that everyone's skin reacts differently. You should test the products on a less sensitive area before using them. You should also remember that even natural products have side effects. The appendix gives the most common expected benefits and results of these ingredients. You should review these entries before trying any recipe.

Grain Scrubs

I love to have a handful of grains available to scrub my face and body every time I shower. I use these scrubs before my soap to remove any surface dirt and oils and to exfoliate my skin in preparation for the remaining treatments in my daily regimen.

You can use many different cleansing grains. The easiest to find and the ones I have found the most effective are:

Uncooked Oatmeal

Cornmeal

Wheat Germ

You may combine these grains or use them individually for great results. Just combine the selected grains with warm distilled water to form a paste. Massage the mixture into your skin with gentle circular motions. Rinse your skin well and follow the treatment with your favorite daily care products.

You can also blend the grains with a cold cream or soap for a foaming action.

Sometimes the loose grains are messy so I use a bag for application. You can make a scrubbing bag out of almost any material but a looser fabric works best. I prefer using muslin cloth cut to size but gauze or cheesecloth squares work well. Mix your favorite grains, grated soap, and oils together in a bowl and spoon the mixture onto your chosen cloth. Tie the cloth closed and you have an excellent rubbing bag for your bath.

While I do add herbs & oils that contain beneficial compounds, I typically do not add color or fragrance to any product designed for damaged skin because additives can cause the irritation to worsen. If you prefer something other than the natural color or scent, you can add your favorite colorant, essential oils, or herbs to the mixture.

Remember that everyone's skin reacts differently. You should test the products on a less sensitive area before using them. You should also remember that even natural products have side effects. The appendix gives the most common expected benefits and results of these ingredients. You should review these entries before trying any recipe.

Fruit Scrubs

Fruit pits & peels contain many of the same benefits and oils as the fruit itself and of the oils extracted from the fruit. I like to have a stronger exfoliation scrub available for more focused care of the rougher patches of my skin such as elbows, knees and feet and for areas that can be prone to extreme outbreaks, like the back.

There are many different fruit pits available in the scrubs sold at your local stores. You can also make your own single or blended fruit pit exfoliation product. You can choose any of the basic fruit pits listed below or experiment with other fruits to see what might work best for your particular needs.

Avocado Pit is very rich in oils that provide exceptional skin softening and conditioning with a more abrasive rubbing action than some other options. Avocado may not be suitable for use in acne care but do a nice job in treatments for seborrhea.

Apricot Kernel contain oils that may be the easiest fruit oil for the skin to absorb. These oils are rich in Vitamin A that is vital for healthy, glowing skin.

Peach Pit is rich in conditioning oils that will aid in keeping skin soft and supple while acting as mild humectant to attract additional moisture to the surface of the skin.

To create a scrub, remove the hard shell from the outside of the pit or seed. Inside the hard shell will be an oil rich nut like product. Grind the nut to the desired consistency.

The larger the finished pieces the more intense the abrasive action of your scrub will be.

For normal skin, grind the pits to a loose powder similar to corn meal in texture. If the skin needs more abrasiveness, grind the pits to a consistency closer to oatmeal. For less abrasive action, powder the pits to a fine dust.

The product will have its own natural scent and color, but if you desire a specific fragrance color to suit your needs or an aromatherapy benefit you may add your favorite colorant or essential oils to the recipe.

While I do add herbs & oils that contain beneficial compounds, I typically do not add color or fragrance to any product designed for damaged skin because additives can cause the irritation to worsen

You can use the scrubs alone or mix them with a cold cream or soap for a foaming action. You may also place your ground pits in a scrubbing bag for easier and cleaner application. Just be sure your chosen bag has large enough mesh to allow the pits abrasive action to come through.

Remember that everyone's skin reacts differently. You should test the products on a less sensitive area before using them. You should also remember that even natural products have side effects. The appendix gives the most common expected benefits and results of these ingredients. You should review these entries before trying any recipe.

Basic Exfoliation Scrub

This is a nice base exfoliation recipe. You can use this recipe as it is written or you can customize this base to suit almost any cleansing need. I try to use this cleanser once or twice a week to help reveal better-looking skin, allow penetration of the compounds of my other cleansing products and improve my skins overall texture.

1 tbsp.	Scrubbing Agent of your choice
	Almonds Powder (rougher skin)
	Oatmeal or Cornmeal (gentle cleansing)
	Ground Citrus Peels (clarifying)
1 tbsp.	Rose Water
1 tsp.	Honey
	Emulsifier & Thickener as desired

Mix all of the ingredients in a blender until well blended but not slush.

Store the finished product in a clean container with a tight fitting lid. This mixture may separate so shake it well before each use.

While I do add herbs & oils that contain beneficial compounds, I typically do not add color or fragrance to any product designed for damaged skin because additives can cause the irritation to worsen. This recipe has a fresh clean smell and a light color. The customizations that you use will add color and additional color and fragrance. If you desire a specific color or fragrance, you may add your favorite colorant or essential oils or herbs to the mixture.

Remember that everyone's skin reacts differently. You should test the products on a less sensitive area before using them. You should also remember that even natural products have side effects. The appendix gives the most common expected benefits and results of these ingredients. You should review these entries before trying any recipe.

Toning Scrub

This mildly abrasive scrub works well as a toning agent and is a great option to help exfoliate her skin while achieving a younger, more toned look and feel.

½	Finely Chopped Cucumber and Peel
2 tbsp.	Jojoba Oil
2 tbsp.	Cucumber Juice
1 tsp.	Lemon Juice
1/8 cup	Rose Water
1/8 cup	Witch Hazel
	Emulsifier & Thickener as desired

Mix all of the ingredients in a blender until they are well blended but not slush.

While I do add herbs & oils that contain beneficial compounds, I typically do not add color or fragrance to any product designed for damaged skin because additives can cause the irritation to worsen. If you prefer something other than the natural color or scent, you can add your favorite colorant, essential oils, or herbs to the mixture.

Store the finished product in a clean container with a tight fitting lid. This mixture may separate so shake it well before each use.

Remember that everyone's skin reacts differently. You should test the products on a less sensitive area before using them. You should also remember that even natural products have side effects. The appendix gives the most common expected benefits and results of these ingredients. You should review these entries before trying any recipe.

Daily Clarifying Cleanser for Extremely Oily Skin

This cleanser works well for acne caused primarily by oily skin. It is also a slightly more soothing alternative to some of the other oily skin cleansing options. I like the light abrasion effect of the oatmeal coupled with the soothing action of the cornmeal. I use this cleanser on my body during the summer when sunscreen and oils tend to make my skin a little oilier than normal and more prone to outbreaks.

¼ cup	Cornstarch
¼ cup	Oatmeal
2 tbsp	Witch Hazel
2 tbsp	Lemon Juice
1 tsp	Lavender Oil
2 tbsp	Grapefruit Juice
	Emulsifier & Thickener as desired

Place all of the ingredients in the blender and whip until the oatmeal is finer and the ingredients are well blended.

While I do add herbs & oils that contain beneficial compounds, I typically do not add color or fragrance to any product designed for damaged skin because additives can cause the irritation to worsen. If you prefer something other than the natural color or scent, you can add your favorite colorant, essential oils, or herbs to the mixture.

Spoon the cleanser into a clean container and seal it tightly.

Store the finished product in the refrigerator to extend the shelf life.

To use, scoop a small amount into your hands and massage into your skin with gentle upward motions. Allow the mixture to sit on the skin for 30-60 seconds before rinsing.

Remember that everyone's skin reacts differently. You should test the products on a less sensitive area before using them. You should also remember that even natural products have side effects. The appendix gives the most common expected benefits and results of these ingredients. You should review these entries before trying any recipe.

Mermaid Bath Rub

Mermaids are said to have beautiful, glowing skin. Maybe this is because of the salt water that they call home. This treatment is very popular in the spas of the United States and Europe. The rub gently removes surface dirt and dead skin cells and then leaves the newly revealed skin in a condition where it can easily absorb the beneficial compounds of post-bath treatments. This treatment can cause additional irritation to damaged skin so only use this if your skin is already in good condition or if you have completed a test to make certain you will not have a bad reaction to the scrub.

½ cup	Sea Salt
½ cup	Epsom Salts
½ cup	Apricot Kernel Oil
1 tsp.	Vitamin E Oil

Mix the salts and oils until they are well blended. They will form a thick paste.

The product will have its own natural scent and color, but if you desire a specific color to suit your needs or an aromatherapy benefit you may add your favorite colorant, essential oils or herbs to the recipe.

While I do add herbs & oils that contain beneficial compounds, I typically do not add color or fragrance to any product designed for damaged skin because additives can cause the irritation to worsen.

Spoon the paste into a clean container and seal it tightly.

To use, massage a handful of the paste into your skin starting at the top of your body and working your way toward your feet. This treatment is not recommended for use on the face or neck.

When you reach your feet, rinse your skin well and pat it dry.

Do not use soap following this treatment because it will minimize the effects.

Be very careful because the oils will make your skin and tub very slippery.

Remember that everyone's skin reacts differently. You should test the products on a less sensitive area before using them. You should also remember that even natural products have side effects. The appendix gives the most common expected benefits and results of these ingredients. You should review these entries before trying any recipe.

Citrus Scrub

This scrub has a clean scent and provides moisture to dry, rough skin while gently removing dead cells. I like to use this in combination with some of my other citrus-based products to provide an all over body theme to the day. The peels are rich in oils and anti-oxidants while the juices provide a wonderful clarifying action.

1 tsp.	Lemon Juice
¼ tsp.	Borax Powder
¼ cup	Pineapple Juice
¼ cup	Jojoba Oil
¼ cup	Aloe Vera Gel
1	Orange or Lemon Peel – finely ground

Blend the ingredients until they are well mixed.

The product will have its own natural scent and color, but if you desire a specific color to suit your needs or an aromatherapy benefit you may add your favorite colorant, oils or herbs to the recipe.

While I do add herbs & oils that contain beneficial compounds, I typically do not add color or fragrance to any product designed for damaged skin because additives can cause the irritation to worsen. If you prefer something other than the natural color or scent, you can add your favorite colorant, essential oils, or herbs to the mixture.

Pour the scrub into a clean container and seal it tightly. Store the unused scrub in the refrigerator to extend its shelf life.

To apply, shake the mixture well and massage a handful into your skin.

I like to follow this treatment with a citrus scented lotion for extra conditioning.

Remember that everyone's skin reacts differently. You should test the products on a less sensitive area before using them. You should also remember that even natural products have side effects. The appendix gives the most common expected benefits and results of these ingredients. You should review these entries before trying any recipe.

Blackhead Scrub

Blackheads can be one of the most difficult acne problems to treat. Blackheads tend to take longer to dissolve than whiteheads and can pose a real dilemma when trying to clear an outbreak. This cleanser works well when used in combination with the correct toner and a spot blackhead treatment stick or serum.

½	Small Tomato
¼ cup	Cucumber Juice
1 tsp.	Lemon Juice
2 tsp.	Witch Hazel
1 tsp.	Carline Thistle Oil
	Emulsifier & Thickener as desired

Combine all of ingredients in a blender until they are well mixed.

This is a very loose and liquid cleanser and may be more difficult to apply. You may wish to select a beneficial thickening agent like Arrowroot or Acacia Powder to add to the recipe.

This mixture will have a reddish color and a clean scent. While I do add herbs & oils that contain beneficial compounds, I typically do not add color or fragrance to any product designed for damaged skin because additives can cause the irritation to worsen. If you prefer something other than the natural color or scent, you can add your favorite colorant, essential oils, or herbs to the mixture.

Pour the finished cleanser into a clean container and seal it tightly.

Store the extra cleanser in the refrigerator between uses.

Remember that everyone's skin reacts differently. You should test the products on a less sensitive area before using them. You should also remember that even natural products have side effects. The appendix gives the most common expected benefits and results of these ingredients. You should review these entries before trying any recipe.

CHAPTER 4

Astringents & Toners

Astringents & Toners are an essential element to maintaining healthy skin. They work with your cleansers and scrub to help to keep the skin free of dirt and oils. Astringents & toners are a fantastic choice to help to get rid of the residue that cleansers sometimes leave behind.

Astringents and toners also help to minimize the appearance of pores. You should select astringent and toner recipes that complement your other daily care regimen components. I like to choose a toner to use throughout the day to keep my skin looking and feeling fresh.

Remember that everyone's skin reacts differently. You should test the products on a less sensitive area before using them. You should also remember that even natural products have side effects. The appendix gives the most common expected benefits and results of these ingredients. You should review these entries before trying any recipe.

Basic Astringent

This is a great basic astringent for every day needs. It works very well as the recipe is written but it also makes an excellent base for custom astringent products designed to suit your specific needs.

5 tbsp	Rose Water

You may substitute distilled water if you prefer.

1 tbsp	Witch Hazel
2 tbsp	Vodka
1/8 tsp	Borax Powder

Dissolve the borax power in the rose water. You may need to heat the rose water slightly to help dissolve the borax powder. Do not boil the rose water since this can cause some of the beneficial compound to be destroyed and will result in some evaporation of the rose Water.

Add the vodka & witch hazel to the rosewater and stir the mixture until it is well blended.

You may want to select ingredients from the appendix to strengthen the affect of the toner. You should decide what ingredients best suit your skin care goals and add them accordingly. You do not have to add any other compounds if you do not need enhanced treatments since this toner works very well alone.

While I do add herbs & oils that contain beneficial compounds, I typically do not add color or fragrance to any product designed for damaged skin because additives can cause the irritation to worsen. If you prefer something other than the natural color or scent, you can add your favorite colorant, essential oils, or herbs to the mixture.

Store the finished toner in an airtight container to prevent evaporation. Apply the toner to your skin using a clean cotton ball. Do not rinse this recipe from your skin. Allow the liquid to dry naturally and continue to work throughout the day. You can use moisturizer & makeup after the liquid has dried.

Remember that everyone's skin reacts differently. You should test the products on a less sensitive area before using them. You should also remember that even natural products have side effects. The appendix gives the most common expected benefits and results of these ingredients. You should review these entries before trying any recipe.

Acne Reducing Toner

This is a gentle and effective all purpose toner. It helps to reduce the appearance of pores while combating the most common causes of acne outbreaks.

½ cup	Witch Hazel
5 drops	Lemongrass Oil
5 drops	Sea Buckthorn Oil

Mix the ingredients in a spritz bottle.

While I do add herbs & oils that contain beneficial compounds, I typically do not add color or fragrance to any product designed for damaged skin because additives can cause the irritation to worsen. If you prefer something other than the natural color or scent, you can add your favorite colorant, essential oils, or herbs to the mixture.

Store the finished toner in a clean container with a tight fitting lid. This mixture will separate when it is left standing so shake well before each use. Spray the toner on the affected area 3-4 times a day. Do not rinse this recipe from your skin. Allow the liquid to dry naturally and continue to work throughout the day. You can use moisturizer & makeup after the liquid has dried.

Remember that everyone's skin reacts differently. You should test the products on a less sensitive area before using them. You should also remember that even natural products have side effects. The appendix gives the most common expected benefits and results of these ingredients. You should review these entries before trying any recipe.

Moisturizing Astringent

Juices from apples, cherries, plums or berries contain natural humectants that attract moisture and provide a smooth texture to the skin. This is one of my favorite astringent products because it helps to keep my skin fresh and combats outbreaks while promoting a nice smooth, tight texture.

½ cup	Juice of Choice
3 tbsp	Rose Water
3 tbsp	Witch Hazel

Pour the ingredients directly into the airtight storage container. Shake the mixture well to blend all of the ingredients.

While I do add herbs & oils that contain beneficial compounds, I typically do not add color or fragrance to any product designed for damaged skin because additives can cause the irritation to worsen. If you prefer something other than the natural color or scent, you can add your favorite colorant, essential oils, or herbs to the mixture.

This recipe may separate so shake it well before each use. You may wish to store this recipe in the refrigerator to extend the shelf life. Do not rinse this recipe from your skin. Allow the liquid to dry naturally and continue to work throughout the day. You can use moisturizer & makeup after the liquid has dried.

Remember that everyone's skin reacts differently. You should test the products on a less sensitive area before using them. You should also remember that even natural products have side effects. The appendix gives the most common expected benefits and results of these ingredients. You should review these entries before trying any recipe.

Wake Up Toner

This is an excellent toner to help wake up dull skin, speed healing, and minimize the appearance of outbreaks. It works equally well on the face and body.

1 cup	Distilled Water
½ tsp.	American Elder Flowers
½ tsp.	Basil Leaves
½ cup	Witch Hazel

Bring the water to a light boil and remove it from the heat. Add the flowers and leaves to the hot water. Steep the flowers & leaves in the water for up to 24 hours or until you achieve a nice dark brew. Strain the flowers and leaves from the fluid and discard the plant parts. The fluid will act as the base for your toner.

Stir witch hazel into the liquid base.

While I do add herbs & oils that contain beneficial compounds, I typically do not add color or fragrance to any product designed for damaged skin because additives can cause the irritation to worsen. If you prefer something other than the natural color or scent, you can add your favorite colorant, essential oils, or herbs to the mixture.

Pour the finished toner into your favorite spray or dispenser bottle. Seal the container tightly to prevent evaporation.

Apply the finished product to your skin using a cotton ball or spritzer.

Do not rinse this recipe from your skin. Allow the liquid to dry naturally and continue to work throughout the day. You can use moisturizer & makeup after the liquid has dried.

Remember that everyone's skin reacts differently. You should test the products on a less sensitive area before using them. You should also remember that even natural products have side effects. The appendix gives the most common expected benefits and results of these ingredients. You should review these entries before trying any recipe

Healing Toner

Honey is one of my favorite skin care ingredients. It not only helps to soften the skin, it also has antibacterial and healing properties. This toner works well for anyone who has skin irritation and helps to combat acne aggravated by bacterial infections.

2 tbsp	Honey
4 tbsp	Strong Chamomile Tea
4 tbsp	Rose Water

You can make the chamomile tea using 1 tbsp. of chamomile and ½ cup water. Bring the water to a boil and then remove it from the heat. Add the chamomile. Allow the mixture to steep up to 24 hours or until a strong tea has been created. Strain the plant parts from the fluid.

Blend all of the ingredients directly into the container you will use as a dispenser.

While I do add herbs & oils that contain beneficial compounds, I typically do not add color or fragrance to any product designed for damaged skin because additives can cause the irritation to worsen. If you prefer something other than the natural color or scent, you can add your favorite colorant, essential oils, or herbs to the mixture.

The toner will be sticky at first. Aging helps to diminish the sticky quality. I like to age this toner for about 1 week before use but you can use it immediately if you wish.

Do not rinse this recipe from your skin. Allow the liquid to dry naturally and continue to work throughout the day. You can use moisturizer & makeup after the liquid has dried.

Remember that everyone's skin reacts differently. You should test the products on a less sensitive area before using them. You should also remember that even natural products have side effects. The appendix gives the most common expected benefits and results of these ingredients. You should review these entries before trying any recipe.

Cooling Toner

Cucumber juice is one of my favorite astringent products. It helps to relieve sore skin, sooth inflammation and speed healing while reducing puffiness. This toner has one of the cleanest scents and is a favorite of everyone in the house.

½ cup	Cucumber Juice
4 tbsp	Witch Hazel
2 tbsp	Rose Water

You can make cucumber juice by chopping the cucumber, including the peel into smaller pieces. Place the pieces into the blender and whip on a medium setting until the pieces are pulped. Strain off the green juice for use in the recipe.

Add the remaining ingredients to the cucumber juice and mix until they are well blended.

While I do add herbs & oils that contain beneficial compounds, I typically do not add color or fragrance to any product designed for damaged skin because additives can cause the irritation to worsen. If you prefer something other than the natural color or scent, you can add your favorite colorant, essential oils, or herbs to the mixture.

Store the completed toner in an airtight container. You may wish to place the container in the refrigerator to increase the shelf life of the finished product.

Do not rinse this recipe from your skin. Allow the liquid to dry naturally and continue to work throughout the day. You can use moisturizer & makeup after the liquid has dried.

Remember that everyone's skin reacts differently. You should test the products on a less sensitive area before using them. You should also remember that even natural products have side effects. The appendix gives the most common expected benefits and results of these ingredients. You should review these entries before trying any recipe.

Restorative Toner

This nice restorative toner helps to speed healing, combat bacteria, and promote clear skin. It is a nice toning choice for those whose skin is fatigued and for use by acne sufferers whose skin is beginning to age.

1 tsp	Honey
1 tsp	Finely Ground Immortelle
¼ cup	Aloe Vera Gel
¼ cup	Witch Hazel

Whip the ingredients until they are well blended.

While I do add herbs & oils that contain beneficial compounds, I typically do not add color or fragrance to any product designed for damaged skin because additives can cause the irritation to worsen. If you prefer something other than the natural color or scent, you can add your favorite colorant, essential oils, or herbs to the mixture.

Store the completed toner in an airtight container.

The toner will be sticky at first. Aging helps to diminish the sticky quality. I like to age this toner about 1 week before use but you can use it immediately you wish.

Do not rinse this recipe from your skin. Allow the liquid to dry naturally and continue to work throughout the day. You can use moisturizer & makeup after the liquid has dried.

Remember that everyone's skin reacts differently. You should test the products on a less sensitive area before using them. You should also remember that even natural products have side effects. The appendix gives the most common expected benefits and results of these ingredients. You should review these entries before trying any recipe.

Gentle Astringent for Sensitive Skin

Having both acne and sensitive skin can cause a major dilemma. Many of the more common acne treatments are harsh and can damage sensitive skin. This nice toner helps to promote clear, fresh looking skin without creating irritation.

4 tbsp   Rose Water

4 tbsp   Orange Flower Distilled Water

Pour the liquids directly into a spray bottle. Shake the bottle well to blend the ingredients.

While I do add herbs & oils that contain beneficial compounds, I typically do not add color or fragrance to any product designed for damaged skin because additives can cause the irritation to worsen. If you prefer something other than the natural color or scent, you can add your favorite colorant, essential oils, or herbs to the mixture.

Shake the completed toner well before each use. Do not rinse this recipe from your skin. Allow the liquid to dry naturally and continue to work throughout the day. You can use moisturizer & makeup after the liquid has dried.

Remember that everyone's skin reacts differently. You should test the products on a less sensitive area before using them. You should also remember that even natural products have side effects. The appendix gives the most common expected benefits and results of these ingredients. You should review these entries before trying any recipe.

Scar Reduction Toner

Sometimes, acne leaves long term pigmentation scars behind. This is a nice toner to use on a regular basis to help reduce the appearance of light pitting and hyper-pigmentation while keeping the skin free of dirt, oils, and toxins.

4 tbsp   Rose Water

4 tbsp   Powdered Avens

Pour the liquids directly into a spray bottle.

While I do add herbs & oils that contain beneficial compounds, I typically do not add color or fragrance to any product designed for damaged skin because additives can cause the irritation to worsen. If you prefer something other than the natural color or scent, you can add your favorite colorant, essential oils, or herbs to the mixture.

Shake the completed toner well before each use. Do not rinse this recipe from your skin. Allow the liquid to dry naturally and continue to work throughout the day. You can use moisturizer & makeup after the liquid has dried.

Remember that everyone's skin reacts differently. You should test the products on a less sensitive area before using them. You should also remember that even natural products have side effects. The appendix gives the most common expected benefits and results of these ingredients. You should review these entries before trying any recipe.

CHAPTER 5

Deep Bath Treatments & Masks

Sometimes a deep treatment helps to maximize the benefits of daily care. At other times, deep treatments are necessary to start the healing processes and remove obstacles that can interfere with your selected daily cleansing & moisturizing plans.

Deep treatments are designed to deliver concentrated benefits to a specific area helping to achieve results much more quickly. Deep treatments should not be overused since they tend to be more concentrated and overuse can actually cause more damage than benefit.

Deep treatments provide an excellent opportunity for you to try your hand at customization with the ingredients in the appendix. Masks & deep treatments help to pamper your skin and prepare it for a daily regimen that will aid you in achieving healthy, blemish-free skin. You should refer to the optional ingredient list to customize the deep treatment recipe, making one that suits your personal needs & desires.

While I do add herbs & oils that contain beneficial compounds, I typically do not add color or fragrance to any product designed for damaged skin because additives can cause the irritation to worsen. If you prefer something other than the natural color or scent, you can add your favorite colorant, essential oils, or herbs to the recipes.

Remember that everyone's skin reacts differently. You should test the products on a less sensitive area before using them. You should also remember that even natural products have side effects. The appendix gives the most common expected benefits and results of these ingredients. You should review these entries before trying any recipe.

Skin Clarifying Soak

Sometimes the root of an acne breakout is a concentration of built up dead skin and oils. Using a deep-treatment clarifying product once or twice a week or even once a month helps to reduce the amount of surface dirt, oils, & toxins that remain on your skin despite your daily regimen. This soak is one of my favorites because it leaves the skin hydrated & healthy while giving me the full body treatment I need to help my daily care regimen work at its best.

¼ cup	Vinegar
1 cup	Orange Flower Distilled Water
½ cup	Rose Water
¼ cup	Sea Salts

Dissolve the salts in the liquid base and shake solution until well blended.

The recipe will have a stronger vinegar smell so you may want to add your favorite fragrances to your solution to alter the smell.

Food coloring may also be added to provide a pretty color to your recipe and your bath Distilled Water. The vinegar smell will fade from your skin very quickly so scent is not necessary to the recipe.

While I do add herbs & oils that contain beneficial compounds, I typically do not add color or fragrance to any product designed for damaged skin because additives can cause the irritation to worsen. If you prefer something other than the natural color or scent, you can add your favorite colorant, essential oils, or herbs to the mixture.

Pour the finished product into a clean container and seal tightly.

You will want to shake the solution before using to ensure the ingredients are well blended.

To use add approximately ¼ cup of the mixture to your bath and soak approximately 15-20 minutes.

If your skin is not oily, you should follow this treatment with a light moisturizer.

Remember that everyone's skin reacts differently. You should test the products on a less sensitive area before using them. You should also remember that even natural products have side effects. The appendix gives the most common expected benefits and results of these ingredients. You should review these entries before trying any recipe.

Simple Hydrating Bath

When treating acne, it is easy to forget that healthy skin is important to blemish free skin. Well-hydrated skin will be better able to absorb the daily treatments, resist scarring more effectively, and look healthier.

1 tbsp.	Chamomile Leaves
1 tbsp.	Basil Leaves
1 cup	Boiling Distilled Water

Bring the water to a light boil and remove it from the heat. Pour the boiling water over the leaves and allow the mixture to steep overnight.

Strain the leaves from the fluid. Add

¼ cup	Carrot Juice
¼ cup	Tomato Juice (without seeds)

Stir the mixture until the ingredients are well blended.

Your recipe will be an orange tone and have a slight aroma. If you wish, you can use colorants, herbs, or oils to alter the color or fragrance.

While I do add herbs & oils that contain beneficial compounds, I typically do not add color or fragrance to any product designed for damaged skin because additives can cause the irritation to worsen. If you prefer something other than the natural color or scent, you can add your favorite colorant, essential oils, or herbs to the mixture.

Pour the finished mixture into your favorite tightly sealed container.

To use, pour ½ of the mixture into a warm bath and soak 15-20 minutes.

Remember that everyone's skin reacts differently. You should test the products on a less sensitive area before using them. You should also remember that even natural products have side effects. The appendix gives the most common expected benefits and results of these ingredients. You should review these entries before trying any recipe.

Skin Soothing Soak

This is an excellent choice for use when skin is irritated and sensitive. This soak helps to relax your mind minimizing the stress that can sometimes contribute to acne outbreaks. The soak also combats bacteria on the skins surface and leaves the skin feeling silky.

¼ cup	Aloe Vera Gel
¼ cup	Epsom Salts
4 tbsp.	Lavender Oil
¼ cup	Apple Juice
¼ cup	Witch Hazel

Dissolve the salts in the witch hazel base.

Add the remaining ingredients and stir until they are well blended.

Pour the finished mixture into a clean container and seal it tightly.

Part of the benefit of this treatment comes from the scent released from the lavender oils. Some acne outbreaks are believed to be caused by stress. Lavender is both anti-bacterial and nervine making it a choice ingredient for treating acne. If you desire the skin benefits without the sedative and relaxing qualities of the lavender aroma, you may exchange the lavender with your favorite scent.

Food coloring may also be added at this time to create a pretty color to your recipe and the bath water.

While I do add herbs & oils that contain beneficial compounds, I typically do not add color or fragrance to any product designed for damaged skin because additives can cause the irritation to worsen.

This mixture may separate if left standing so you should shake the mixture well before each use.

To use, add approximately ¼ cup to warm bath water and soak for 10-15 minutes or until the desired soothing effect has been achieved.

Remember that everyone's skin reacts differently. You should test the products on a less sensitive area before using them. You should also remember that even natural products have side effects. The appendix gives the most common expected benefits and results of these ingredients. You should review these entries before trying any recipe.

Cleansing Bubble Bath

The basic bubble bath formula helps to clean & hydrate the skin while eliminating bacteria. The innate scent of the bath is wonderful & refreshing

¼ cup	Liquid Castile Soap
1 tsp.	Honey Powder
1 tsp.	Tea Tree Oil
1 tbsp.	Jojoba Oil
2 tbsp.	Coconut Oil

Combine the ingredients and gently mix until they are well blended. Do not whip the mixture since it will foam.

While I do add herbs & oils that contain beneficial compounds, I typically do not add color or fragrance to any product designed for damaged skin because additives can cause the irritation to worsen. If you prefer something other than the natural color or scent, you can add your favorite colorant, essential oils, or herbs to the mixture.

Pour the completed mixture into tightly sealed container.

To use, pour a small amount of the cleanser under the running water as you fill your bath.

Remember that everyone's skin reacts differently. You should test the products on a less sensitive area before using them. You should also remember that even natural products have side effects. The appendix gives the most common expected benefits and results of these ingredients. You should review these entries before trying any recipe.

Soothing Salts

This excellent bath salt helps to pamper the skin. It works well as a bath soak additive or scrub that helps to sooth and hydrate while combating both tension & bacteria that can contribute to an acne outbreak.

1 cup   Epsom Salts

1 cup   Uncooked Oatmeal

2 tsp.   Tea Tree Oil

1 tsp.   Lavender Oil

Combine the dry ingredients in a container.

Pour the oils over the mixture and shake it until the oils are evenly distributed.

While I do add herbs & oils that contain beneficial compounds, I typically do not add color or fragrance to any product designed for damaged skin because additives can cause the irritation to worsen. If you prefer something other than the natural color or scent, you can add your favorite colorant, essential oils, or herbs to the mixture.

To add a fragrance or color sprinkle the desired item over the mixture similar to the way you mixed in the oils.

Shake the salts to distribute the color or fragrance and seal the container tightly.

To use pour approximately ¼ cup in the warm bath water or rub a handful of the mixture over the skin for a nice shower or bath scrub.

Remember that everyone's skin reacts differently. You should test the products on a less sensitive area before using them. You should also remember that even natural products have side effects. The appendix gives the most common expected benefits and results of these ingredients. You should review these entries before trying any recipe.

Ivy Bath Soak

English Ivy is an excellent product for use when getting your skin ready for special occasions. The ivy helps draw fluids from the skin and reduces the appearance of acne, water retention, and other unsightly conditions. This mixture will tighten and tone the skin leaving it looking and feeling wonderful. You should not use this recipe for facial products.

10	English Ivy Leaves
½ cup	Distilled Water

Heat the water to a light boil and remove it from the heat. Pour the heated water over the ivy leaves and allow the mixture to soak for 24 hours. Strain the leaves from the water and discard them. The fluid will act as the base for your recipe.

¼ cup	Jojoba Oil
3 tbsp.	Seaweed Powder

Add the oil and powder to your ivy Distilled Water and blend ingredients until they are well mixed.

While I do add herbs & oils that contain beneficial compounds, I typically do not add color or fragrance to any product designed for damaged skin because additives can cause the irritation to worsen. If you prefer something other than the natural color or scent, you can add your favorite colorant, essential oils, or herbs to the mixture.

Pour the completed solution into clean container and seal it tightly.

To use, shake the mixture well and pour ¼ cup into your bath. Soak for 20-30 minutes. Follow the treatment with a hydrating and toning moisturizer for the best effect.

Remember that everyone's skin reacts differently. You should test the products on a less sensitive area before using them. You should also remember that even natural products have side effects. The appendix gives the most common expected benefits and results of these ingredients. You should review these entries before trying any recipe.

Nighttime Bath for Damaged Skin

This is an excellent balm for irritated or injured skin. I keep this mixed and available to use whenever my skin needs some extra special care.

¼ cup	Dried Basil
½ cup	Distilled Water

Bring the water to a boil and remove it from the heat. Pour the water over the basil and allow solution to steep 24 hours. Strain the basil from the water and discard the leaves. The fluid will be the base for the recipe.

2 tbsp.	Hazelnut Oil
2 tbsp.	Macadamia Nut Oil
1 tbsp.	Glycerin
2 tbsp.	Honey Powder
3 tbsp.	Aloe Vera Gel

Combine the remaining ingredients with the basil water stirring until they are well blended.

The mixture will have a wonderful aroma from the ingredients. While I do add herbs & oils that contain beneficial compounds, I typically do not add color or fragrance to any product designed for damaged skin because additives can cause the irritation to worsen. If you prefer something other than the natural color or scent, you can add your favorite colorant, essential oils, or herbs to the mixture.

Pour the finished mixture into a container and seal it tightly.

To use the bath, add ¼ cup of the liquid to your warm bath Distilled Water and soak until relief is obtained or 20-30 minutes.

You may need to repeat the process if the skin is especially irritated or sore.

For the best affect, follow the treatment with a soothing & healing moisturizer.

Remember that everyone's skin reacts differently. You should test the products on a less sensitive area before using them. You should also remember that even natural products have side effects. The appendix gives the most common expected benefits and results of these ingredients. You should review these entries before trying any recipe.

Foaming Bath Gel

I love using this gel in my bath when I know that my skin will be exposed to environmental factors that might contribute to an outbreak. The mixture has an excellent foaming effect that provides a moisturizing, protecting film to your skin. It works especially well for chapped, irritated, or dehydrated skin.

1 tbsp.   Grated Beeswax

½ cup   Jojoba Oil

Heat beeswax and oil in the microwave in a microwave safe dish or in a double broiler until it reaches approximately 90 degrees. Remove the oil from the heat and add

3 tsp.   Borax Powder

2 tbsp.   Honey

Mix the remaining ingredients with the heated oils until well blended.

While I do add herbs & oils that contain beneficial compounds, I typically do not add color or fragrance to any product designed for damaged skin because additives can cause the irritation to worsen. If you prefer something other than the natural color or scent, you can add your favorite colorant, essential oils, or herbs to the mixture.

Pour the completed mixture into a pump container.

To use, pump one or two squirts into the palm of your hand and apply directly to the skin or into the running bath water.

The oils that remain on the skin after your bath will provide a moisturizing, protective film.

The tub may be slippery and should be cleaned thoroughly after the treatment.

Remember that everyone's skin reacts differently. You should test the products on a less sensitive area before using them. You should also remember that even natural products have side effects. The appendix gives the most common expected benefits and results of these ingredients. You should review these entries before trying any recipe.

Skin Renewal Body Mask

This body-mask is very popular in day spas. The mask extracts toxins from below the surface of the skin and leaves a beautiful clear glow behind. I love to use this recipe at least once a month to keep my skin clear.

½ cup	Powdered Clay
¼ cup	Powdered Kelp (seaweed)
2 tbsp.	Sea Salt
¼ cup	Distilled Water
3 tbsp.	Jojoba Oil
¼ cup	Aloe Vera Gel

Blend the water and oil with the sea salt and powdered kelp. Whip the aloe vera gel into the mixture.

Stir until the powder and salts are dissolved.

Slowly add the clay powder until a thick paste is formed and all of the ingredients are moist and well mixed.

If the powder is too dry and flaky, add small amounts of distilled water until the correct texture is achieved.

The product will have its own natural scent and color, but if you desire a specific color to suit your needs or an aromatherapy benefit you may add your favorite colorant or essential oils to the recipe. I typically do not add color or fragrance to any product designed for damaged skin because additives can cause the irritation to worsen.

Spread the clay mixture all over your body. I like to use a sea sponge to spread the mixture but you may use any applicator you wish.

Allow the mask to dry and harden – approximately 15-20 minutes. Rinse the clay from your body and pat the skin dry. I typically follow this treatment with a moisture rich lotion.

Remember that everyone's skin reacts differently. You should test the products on a less sensitive area before using them. You should also remember that even natural products have side effects. The appendix gives the most common expected benefits and results of these ingredients. You should review these entries before trying any recipe.

Steam Treatment

One of the most effective daily treatments for clear, healthy looking skin is a steam treatment.

There are many machines available for steam treatments but they are not necessary for using steam & herbs to help open your pores and clean your skin.

You can use a stainless steel or other pot that does not have a coating that will release chemicals into the liquid as it boils.

2 cups	Distilled Water
1 tsp.	Bay Leaves
1 tsp.	Spearmint Leaves

You can add the herbs loose or use a tea ball to contain the plant parts.

Place a clean, cotton towel over the top of the pan.

Bring the water & herb mixture to a light boil.

Gently lift the edge of the towel to direct the steam.

Use your hand to test the temperature of the steam before putting your face into the flow. Your hand will help you to find the distance that gives you warm but not hot steam.

Place your face in the stream of steam.

Relax and allow the moisture and plant compounds to do their job.

When you are finished, rinse your face with cool Distilled Water and gently pat it dry.

Kelp Treatment

This nice deep cleansing treatment literally allows you to peel away toxins and build up that can cause acne.

3 tbsp.   Powdered Brown Kelp

2 tbsp.   Powdered Raspberry Leaves

8 tbsp.   Rose Water

Dissolve the powders in the rose water. If the mask is too solid, add a few extra drops of rose water. If the mask is too liquid, add a few sprinkles of powdered kelp.

The product will have its own natural scent and color, but if you desire a specific color to suit your needs or an aromatherapy benefit you may add your favorite colorant or essential oils to the recipe. While I do add herbs & oils that contain beneficial compounds, I typically do not add color or fragrance to any product designed for damaged skin because additives can cause the irritation to worsen.

To use, apply the paste to your skin in an even coat.

Allow the mixture to soak into your skin for approximately 30 minutes or until it is completely dry.

Peel the mixture from the skin, rinse well, and pat the skin dry.

Remember that everyone's skin reacts differently. You should test the products on a less sensitive area before using them. You should also remember that even natural products have side effects. The appendix gives the most common expected benefits and results of these ingredients. You should review these entries before trying any recipe.

Gelatin Toning Mask or Wrap

Gelatin is one of my favorite mask bases. It is not as drawing as clay but it does help to attract moisture to the skin. My skin can get irritated when I use too many products too close together. This helps minimize the irritation while minimizing the duration and severity of an attack.

½ cup   Gelatin – 1 packet

½ cup   Warm Distilled Water

½ tsp.   Lemon Juice

½ tsp.   Bergamot

Mix the gelatin and water until they are well blended.

Before the gelatin hardens, stir in the remaining ingredients.

The product will have its own natural scent and color, but if you desire a specific color to suit your needs or an aromatherapy benefit you may add your favorite colorant or essential oils to the recipe. While I do add herbs & oils that contain beneficial compounds, I typically do not add color or fragrance to any product designed for damaged skin because additives can cause the irritation to worsen.

To use, apply the mixture to your skin in an even coat.

Allow the mixture to soak into your skin for approximately 30 minutes or until the gelatin is completely dry.

Peel or rinse the mask from your skin.

Remember that everyone's skin reacts differently. You should test the products on a less sensitive area before using them. You should also remember that even natural products have side effects. The appendix gives the most common expected benefits and results of these ingredients. You should review these entries before trying any recipe.

Clear Skin Wrap

This body wrap is a one of my favorite recipes. It actually helps to reduce the appearance of acne while toning the skin.

½ cup	Powdered Clay
¼ cup	Radish Juice
¼ cup	Warm Distilled Water
10	Finely Ground English Ivy Leaves
1 tbsp.	Palmaris Oil
2 tbsp.	Sea Salt

Mix the juice and the water with the oil.

Dissolve the sea salt in the liquid solution and then add the ivy powder.

Slowly add the clay powder until a thick paste is formed. You do not want the mixture to be too wet since it may be difficult to apply. If it is too wet, add a bit more clay. If the mixture is too firm, you can add a few drops of water until you get the consistency you want.

The product will have its own natural scent and color, but if you desire a specific color to suit your needs or an aromatherapy benefit you may add your favorite colorant or essential oils to the recipe. While I do add herbs & oils that contain beneficial compounds, I typically do not add color or fragrance to any product designed for damaged skin because additives can cause the irritation to worsen.

To use, apply the mixture to your skin in an even coat.

Allow the mixture to soak into your skin for approximately 30 minutes or until the wrap is completely dry.

Rinse the wrap from your skin and follow the treatment with a toning moisturizer.

Remember that everyone's skin reacts differently. You should test the products on a less sensitive area before using them. You should also remember that even natural products have side effects. The appendix gives the most common expected benefits and results of these ingredients. You should review these entries before trying any recipe.

Aloe Vera Healing Wrap

Aloe Vera is a wonderful treatment for many, many problems. Perhaps one of the best uses is for the treatment of acne outbreaks. Aloe helps to reduce bacteria while speeding healing and soothing irritation. Goldenseal and Agrimony are two of my favorite additives for use with acne care but you can select almost any other powder or oil from the appendix list to include in your personal healing wrap.

¼ cup	Powdered Clay – Kaolin works best
¼ cup	Aloe Vera Gel
1 tbsp.	Powdered Agrimony
1 tbsp.	Powdered Goldenseal

Blend the dry ingredients and slowly add them to the aloe vera base until a thick paste is formed.

The product will have its own natural scent and color, but if you desire a specific color to suit your needs or an aromatherapy benefit you may add your favorite colorant or essential oils to the recipe. While I do add herbs & oils that contain beneficial compounds, I typically do not add color or fragrance to any product designed for damaged skin because additives can cause the irritation to worsen.

To use, apply the mixture to your skin in an even coat.

Allow the mixture to soak into your skin for approximately 30 minutes or until the gelatin is completely dry.

Rinse the wrap from your skin and follow it with a healing moisturizing treatment.

Remember that everyone's skin reacts differently. You should test the products on a less sensitive area before using them. You should also remember that even natural products have side effects. The appendix gives the most common expected benefits and results of these ingredients. You should review these entries before trying any recipe.

Henna Wrap

Henna helps to ease the discomfort and appearance of acne and seborrhea. This wrap is packed with acne healing ingredients and is one of the nicest choices for easing a severe outbreak. Henna comes in colored and colorless forms and you will want to be sure that you are using colorless henna powder unless you are hoping to make a sunless tanning product out of your wrap!

½ cup   Colorless Henna Powder

¼ cup   Witch Hazel

¼ cup   Warm Distilled Water

2 tbsp.   Powdered Lemongrass

Stir the lemongrass and henna powders until they are well blended.

Slowly add the blended powders to the liquid until the ingredients form a thick paste. If the mixture is too liquid, you can add a bit more henna powder. If the mixture it too solid, you can add a few extra drops of witch hazel.

The product will have its own natural scent and color, but if you desire a specific color to suit your needs or an aromatherapy benefit you may add your favorite colorant or essential oils to the recipe. While I do add herbs & oils that contain beneficial compounds, I typically do not add color or fragrance to any product designed for damaged skin because additives can cause the irritation to worsen.

To use, apply the mixture to your skin in an even coat.

Allow the mixture to soak into your skin for approximately 30 minutes or until the gelatin is completely dry.

Rinse the mask from your skin and follow with a hydrating moisturizer.

Remember that everyone's skin reacts differently. You should test the products on a less sensitive area before using them. You should also remember that even natural products have side effects. The appendix gives the most common expected benefits and results of these ingredients. You should review these entries before trying any recipe.

CHAPTER 6

Sticks, Serums, & Lotions

Healthy skin is not just about cleansing. Healthy skin is about creating the right mixture of cleanliness, hydration, and moisture. Serums & lotions are critical to the success of your skin care regimen.

Your skin may need additional serums and treatments to help combat the dryness created by other treatments, target specific outbreak problems, and speed the healing process. Serums tend to be lightweight and thinner making applications to the face, neck, and smaller areas easier.

Lotions work much like serums but are traditionally thicker and heavier. While serums work well on the face, lotions tend to be a better choice for the body.

Spot treatments are localized treatments that you can apply directly to the eruption. Serums can be spread over larger areas of skin but tend to be more concentrated so they should be used somewhat sparingly. Lotions are meant for treating large areas of skin over a period of time. Both products help to speed healing, minimize future outbreaks, and reduce the appearance of current outbreaks.

Remember that everyone's skin reacts differently. You should test the products on a less sensitive area before using them. You should also remember that even natural products have side effects. The appendix gives the most common expected benefits and results of these ingredients. You should review these entries before trying any recipe.

Lip Blemish Sticks

At times, we all get a pimple, ulcer, or other blemish around our lip area. Lips can be one of the hardest places to treat. This blemish stick will help to promote faster healing of these eruptions while aiding in the prevention of additional blemishes. This stick can be used on other areas of the body as well.

4 tbsp.	Grated Beeswax
1 tsp.	Honey
2 tbsp.	Juniper Oil
1 tsp.	Powdered Clove
1	Vitamin C Tablet
	Flavors, Colors, Emulsifier & Thickener as desired

Place the beeswax and honey in a microwave safe dish and heat on medium approximately 25 seconds or use a double broiler to liquefy the ingredients bringing them to about 90 degrees Fahrenheit. Remove the mixture from the heat and allow it to cool to approximately 70 degrees.

Add the juniper oil to the cooling mixture.

Dissolve the crushed Vitamin C tablet in the heated solution and blend it well.

While I do add herbs & oils that contain beneficial compounds, I typically do not add color or fragrance to any product designed for damaged skin because additives can cause the irritation to worsen. If you prefer something other than the natural color or scent, you can add your favorite colorant, essential oils, or herbs to the mixture.

Pour the mixture into a greased pan and place it in a cool area. It will harden over 12-16 hours. You may place the container in the refrigerator for faster results.

Cut the hardened mixture into sticks and apply to blemishes as needed.

Remember that everyone's skin reacts differently. You should test the products on a less sensitive area before using them. You should also remember that even natural products have side effects. The appendix gives the most common expected benefits and results of these ingredients. You should review these entries before trying any recipe.

General Blemish Sticks

These are nice sticks to carry with you for spot treatments throughout the day. I like to apply a thin film over current outbreaks every few hours to help reduce redness and speed healing.

4 tbsp.	Grated Beeswax
1 tsp.	Honey
½ tsp.	Caje Oil
½ tsp.	Camphor Oil
1	Vitamin C Tablet
	Flavors, Colors, Emulsifier & Thickener as desired

Place the beeswax and honey in a microwave safe dish and heat on medium approximately 25 seconds or use a double broiler to liquefy the ingredients bringing them to approximately 90 degrees Fahrenheit. Remove the mixture from the heat and allow it to cool to approximately 70 degrees.

Add the oils to the cooling mixture.

Dissolve the crushed Vitamin C tablet in the heated solution and mix well.

While I do add herbs & oils that contain beneficial compounds, I typically do not add color or fragrance to any product designed for damaged skin because additives can cause the irritation to worsen. If you prefer something other than the natural color or scent, you can add your favorite colorant, essential oils, or herbs to the mixture.

Pour the mixture into a greased pan and place it in a cool area. It will harden over 12-16 hours. You may place the container in the refrigerator for faster results.

Cut the hardened mixture into sticks and apply to blemishes as needed.

Remember that everyone's skin reacts differently. You should test the products on a less sensitive area before using them. You should also remember that even natural products have side effects. The appendix gives the most common expected benefits and results of these ingredients. You should review these entries before trying any recipe.

Spot Serum

This is a nice spot serum that helps to reduce bacteria & inflammation while speeding healing of current outbreaks.

2 tsp.	Macadamia Nut Oil
4 drops	Patchouli Essential Oil.
½ tsp	Vitamin E Oil
½ tsp	Sea Buckthorn Berry Juice
	Emulsifier & Thickener as desired

Blend all of the oils in a clean container with a tight fitting lid.

While I do add herbs & oils that contain beneficial compounds, I typically do not add color or fragrance to any product designed for damaged skin because additives can cause the irritation to worsen. If you prefer something other than the natural color or scent, you can add your favorite colorant, essential oils, or herbs to the mixture.

The oils may separate if allowed to sit so shake the mixture well before each use. Dab the oils onto the skin that needs treated. Do not rinse the oils from your skin.

Remember that everyone's skin reacts differently. You should test the products on a less sensitive area before using them. You should also remember that even natural products have side effects. The appendix gives the most common expected benefits and results of these ingredients. You should review these entries before trying any recipe.

Soothing Gel

Many of the treatment recipes included in this book help to reduce acne outbreaks but they may also cause irritation and actually worsen the appearance of skin even while the acne is clearing. This is one of my favorite serums to use to help further fight acne outbreaks while soothing and improving the overall appearance of the skin.

2 tsp	Aloe Oil
2 tsp	Angelica Oil
1 tsp.	Argan Oil

Blend the oils in a clean container with a tight fitting lid.

While I do add herbs & oils that contain beneficial compounds, I typically do not add color or fragrance to any product designed for damaged skin because additives can cause the irritation to worsen. If you prefer something other than the natural color or scent, you can add your favorite colorant, essential oils, or herbs to the mixture.

The oils may separate if allowed to sit so shake the mixture well before each use. Apply the mixture to the skin in the morning and at bedtime. Do not rinse the oils from the skin.

Remember that everyone's skin reacts differently. You should test the products on a less sensitive area before using them. You should also remember that even natural products have side effects. The appendix gives the most common expected benefits and results of these ingredients. You should review these entries before trying any recipe.

Acne Clearing Serum

Jojoba is an excellent base for acne treatment creams and serums since it is close to the skins natural oils and easily absorbed. Jojoba also helps to reduce the dried sebum that is at the heart of an acne outbreak. This is my base serum for every day use.

2 tsp.	Jojoba Oil
¼ tsp.	Sweet Gale Oil
¼ tsp.	Bayberry Oil
	Emulsifier & Thickener as desired

While I do add herbs & oils that contain beneficial compounds, I typically do not add color or fragrance to any product designed for damaged skin because additives can cause the irritation to worsen. If you prefer something other than the natural color or scent, you can add your favorite colorant, essential oils, or herbs to the mixture.

Gently blend the oils in a clean container. Store the mixture in a pump container that allows you to dispense 1 or 2 drops at a time. The oils may separate if allowed to sit so shake the mixture well before each use. Apply an even coat of the oils to the skin in the morning and at night. Do not rinse the mixture from the skin.

Remember that everyone's skin reacts differently. You should test the products on a less sensitive area before using them. You should also remember that even natural products have side effects. The appendix gives the most common expected benefits and results of these ingredients. You should review these entries before trying any recipe.

Healing Serum

This serum helps to speed healing while fighting future outbreaks. It also gives a nice, light finish that works well under makeup making it one of my favorite daytime serums. It is especially compatible with mineral makeup applications.

2 tsp.   Hazelnut Oil

2 tsp.   Heartseed Walnut Oil

1 tsp.   Jojoba Oil

While I do add herbs & oils that contain beneficial compounds, I typically do not add color or fragrance to any product designed for damaged skin because additives can cause the irritation to worsen. If you prefer something other than the natural color or scent, you can add your favorite colorant, essential oils, or herbs to the mixture.

Gently blend the oils in a clean container. Store the mixture in a pump container that allows you to dispense 1 or 2 drops at a time. The oils may separate if allowed to sit so shake the mixture well before each use Apply an even coat of the oils to the skin in the morning and at night. Do not rinse the mixture from the skin.

Remember that everyone's skin reacts differently. You should test the products on a less sensitive area before using them. You should also remember that even natural products have side effects. The appendix gives the most common expected benefits and results of these ingredients. You should review these entries before trying any recipe.

Blackhead Serum

This deep penetrating serum works very well at treating blackheads on the face & body. It penetrates deep into the follicles and actually softens the oxidized sebum that causes blackheads to appear on the surface of the skin.

2 tsp.   Kukui Nut Oil

2 tsp.   Jojoba Oil

5 drops   Lavender Oil.

While I do add herbs & oils that contain beneficial compounds, I typically do not add color or fragrance to any product designed for damaged skin because additives can cause the irritation to worsen. If you prefer something other than the natural color or scent, you can add your favorite colorant, essential oils, or herbs to the mixture.

Gently blend the oils in a clean container. Store the mixture in a pump container that allows you to dispense 1 or 2 drops at a time. The oils may separate if allowed to sit so shake the mixture well before each use. Apply an even coat of the oils to the skin in the morning and at night. Do not rinse the mixture from the skin.

Remember that everyone's skin reacts differently. You should test the products on a less sensitive area before using them. You should also remember that even natural products have side effects. The appendix gives the most common expected benefits and results of these ingredients. You should review these entries before trying any recipe.

Pore Reduction Serum

One of the hardest parts of treating acne outbreaks is the enlarged pores some treatments leave behind. This is a nice serum for reducing the appearance of pores while fighting future outbreaks.

2 tsp.   Lemongrass Oil

¼ tsp.   Lime Juice

5 drops   Patchouli Oil

While I do add herbs & oils that contain beneficial compounds, I typically do not add color or fragrance to any product designed for damaged skin because additives can cause the irritation to worsen. If you prefer something other than the natural color or scent, you can add your favorite colorant, essential oils, or herbs to the mixture.

Gently blend the oils in a clean container. Store the mixture in a pump container that allows you to dispense 1 or 2 drops at a time. The oils may separate if allowed to sit so shake the mixture well before each use. Apply an even coat of the oils to the skin in the morning and at night. Do not rinse the mixture from the skin.

Remember that everyone's skin reacts differently. You should test the products on a less sensitive area before using them. You should also remember that even natural products have side effects. The appendix gives the most common expected benefits and results of these ingredients. You should review these entries before trying any recipe.

Hydrating Serum

This wonderful serum helps to reduce the appearance of both seborrhea and acne while hydrating the skin and reducing future outbreaks.

1 tsp	Jojoba Oil
1 tsp	Argan Oil
1 tsp	Immortelle Oil
2 tsp	Sea Buckthorn Oil
	Emulsifier & Thickener as desired

While I do add herbs & oils that contain beneficial compounds, I typically do not add color or fragrance to any product designed for damaged skin because additives can cause the irritation to worsen. If you prefer something other than the natural color or scent, you can add your favorite colorant, essential oils, or herbs to the mixture.

Gently blend the oils in a clean container. Store the mixture in a pump container that allows you to dispense 1 or 2 drops at a time. The oils may separate if allowed to sit so shake the mixture well before each use. Apply an even coat of the oils to the skin in the morning and at night. Do not rinse the mixture from the skin.

Remember that everyone's skin reacts differently. You should test the products on a less sensitive area before using them. You should also remember that even natural products have side effects. The appendix gives the most common expected benefits and results of these ingredients. You should review these entries before trying any recipe.

Basic Acne Serum

This is the most basic of acne treatment serums. It is one that I use to stop an outbreak in its tracks. It also helps to prevent future outbreaks.

¼ cup	Jojoba Oil
1 tsp.	Sandalwood Oil
1 tsp.	Camphor
1 tsp.	Adder's Tongue
1 tsp.	Cypress Oil

While I do add herbs & oils that contain beneficial compounds, I typically do not add color or fragrance to any product designed for damaged skin because additives can cause the irritation to worsen. If you prefer something other than the natural color or scent, you can add your favorite colorant, essential oils, or herbs to the mixture.

Gently blend the oils in a clean container. Store the mixture in a pump container that allows you to dispense 1 or 2 drops at a time. The oils may separate if allowed to sit so shake the mixture well before each use. Apply an even coat of the oils to the skin in the morning and at night. Do not rinse the mixture from the skin. Do not use this serum around the eye area.

Remember that everyone's skin reacts differently. You should test the products on a less sensitive area before using them. You should also remember that even natural products have side effects. The appendix gives the most common expected benefits and results of these ingredients. You should review these entries before trying any recipe.

Protective Lotion

This lotion provides extra skin protection ingredients. I like to use this whenever I have been using a lot specialized treatments that make my skin extra dry & sensitive. The beeswax and oils form a protective layer on the skin making it difficult for dirt and harmful chemicals to cause further damage. This is a great lotion year round for normal to dry acne-prone skin.

2 tbsp.	Grated Beeswax
¼ tsp.	Borax Powder
¼ cup	Jojoba Oil
¼ cup	Tincture of Benzoin
¼ cup	Distilled Water
	Emulsifier & Thickener as desired

Place the beeswax, honey and oil in a microwave safe dish and heat on medium approximately 25 seconds or use a double broiler to liquefy the ingredients bringing them to approximately 90 degrees Fahrenheit.

Remove the mixture from the microwave and set aside to cool slightly to about 70 degrees.

Dissolve the borax powder in the water and heat it until it is just boiling.

Slowly pour the borax solution into the oil and beeswax mixture.

Whip the mixture with a whisk or in a blender until it foams slightly and all ingredients are well blended.

While I do add herbs & oils that contain beneficial compounds, I typically do not add color or fragrance to any product designed for damaged skin because additives can cause the irritation to worsen. If you prefer something other than the natural color or scent, you can add your favorite colorant, essential oils, or herbs to the mixture.

Pour the lotion into a clean container and allow it to cool. The lotion will thicken as it cools.

Remember that everyone's skin reacts differently. You should test the products on a less sensitive area before using them. You should also remember that even natural products have side effects. The appendix gives the most common expected benefits and results of these ingredients. You should review these entries before trying any recipe.

Glowing Daily Lotion

Currently many products on the market provide an unnatural glow to the skin. These products contain everything from crystals to metal. This fantastic lotion will allow your skins natural glow to shine through without creating additional irritation that may lead to an outbreak. I love to use this lotion in the summer months when my skin needs nourishment and I can show off the natural glow that is a part of my skin.

2 tbsp.   Grated Beeswax

1 tbsp.   Palma Rosa Oil

Place the beeswax in a microwave safe dish and heat on medium approximately 25 seconds or use a double broiler to melt the beeswax bringing it to about 90 degrees. Remove the beeswax from the heat and add

¼ cup   Sea Buckthorn

¼ tsp.   Borax Powder

Slowly add the borax mixture to the beeswax syrup.

¼ cup   Aloe Vera Gel

             Emulsifier & Thickener as desired

Add the aloe vera gel to the base mixture and blend the ingredients until they are well mixed.

While I do add herbs & oils that contain beneficial compounds, I typically do not add color or fragrance to any product designed for damaged skin because additives can cause the irritation to worsen. If you prefer something other than the natural color or scent, you can add your favorite colorant, essential oils, or herbs to the mixture.

Pour the lotion into a clean container and allow it to cool completely.

The mixture will thicken as it stands. Tightly seal the container.

Remember that everyone's skin reacts differently. You should test the products on a less sensitive area before using them. You should also remember that even natural products have side effects. The appendix gives the most common expected benefits and results of these ingredients. You should review these entries before trying any recipe.

Pear Lotion for Red Blotchy Skin

This is a great treatment to use anytime environmental factors create havoc with your skin. It also helps to reduce the red, flaky skin associated with seborrhea. I love the soft scent of the pears, but you could use other fruits that contain sorbitol such as apples, cherries, plums or berries. Sorbitol is a natural humectrant that attracts moisture and provides a smooth texture to the skin.

2 tbsp.	Grated Beeswax
2 tbsp.	Jojoba Oil
¼ cup	Sesame Seed Oil
¼ cup	Juice (pear, apple, cherry, plum or berry)
2 tbsp.	Witch Hazel
¼ tsp.	Borax Powder
	Emulsifier & Thickener as desired

Place the beeswax and oils in a microwave safe dish and heat on medium approximately 25 seconds or use a double broiler to liquefy the mixture bringing it to approximately 90 degrees Fahrenheit. Remove the mixture from the heat and allow it to cool to approximately 70 degrees.

Combine the remaining ingredients in another dish.

Heat the witch hazel mixture unit it is hot but not boiling - approximately 35 seconds on medium heat.

Pour the juice mixture into the oil mixture and stir until well blended.

I love the natural smells and colors of this recipe and can alter the final product by changing the type of juice I use.

While I do add herbs & oils that contain beneficial compounds, I typically do not add color or fragrance to any product designed for damaged skin because additives can cause the irritation to worsen. If you prefer something other than the natural color or scent, you can add your favorite colorant, essential oils, or herbs to the mixture.

Allow the recipe to cool before use. The mixture will thicken as it cools.

Remember that everyone's skin reacts differently. You should test the products on a less sensitive area before using them. You should also remember that even natural products have side effects. The appendix gives the most common expected benefits and results of these ingredients. You should review these entries before trying any recipe.

Irritated Skin Balm

This light, non-greasy balm helps to sooth dry or irritated skin. The ingredients soothe the skin and the lavender oils help to calm the nerves and reduce that may contribute to acne outbreaks.

½ cup	Aloe Vera Gel
¼ cup	Apple Juice
1 tbsp.	Witch Hazel
1 tbsp.	Zinc Oxide

2 tsp. Cornstarch

¼ tsp.	Lavender Oil
	Emulsifier & Thickener as desired

Combine the aloe vera gel, apple juice, zinc and witch hazel in a microwave safe dish.

Heat on medium approximately 30 seconds or until it has turned into a liquid or use a double broiler to bring the mixture to approximately 90 degrees Fahrenheit. Remove the mixture from the heat and allow it to cool to approximately 70 degrees.

Add the cornstarch and lavender oil to the cooling mixture.

The product will have its own natural scent and color, but if you desire a specific color to suit your needs or an aromatherapy benefit you may add your favorite colorant or essential oils to the recipe. While I do add herbs & oils that contain beneficial compounds, I typically do not add color or fragrance to any product designed for damaged skin because additives can cause the irritation to worsen. If you prefer something other than the natural color or scent, you can add your favorite colorant, essential oils, or herbs to the mixture.

Pour the mixture into a clean container and allow it to cool completely before use.

This mixture will be a little runnier so you may apply it as usual or use a cotton ball for easier application.

Remember that everyone's skin reacts differently. You should test the products on a less sensitive area before using them. You should also remember that even natural products have side effects. The appendix gives the most common expected benefits and results of these ingredients. You should review these entries before trying any recipe.

Severe Irritation Balm

When skin irritation is a little more severe, you may want to use something a little stronger. This balm should not be used on children and you should consult your physician before using any product if a severe irritation is present. Arrowroot is an anti-inflammatory that helps reduce the swelling that is often present with skin irritation while the other ingredients reduce the pain often associated with acne.

1 tbsp.	Chamomile Leaves
½ cup	Boiling Distilled Water

Heat the water until it is just boiling. Remove the water from the heat and pour it over the chamomile leaves. Allow the mixture to steep at least 6 hours until a darker tea is created. Strain the leaves from the tea and discard them. The liquid will act as your lotion base. Add

1 tbsp.	Arrowroot Powder
1 tsp.	Baking Soda

Dissolve the powders in the tea solution.

1 tbsp.	Jojoba Oil
1 tbsp.	Zinc Oxide
1 tbsp.	Grated Beeswax
1 tbsp.	Neem Oil
	Emulsifier & Thickener as desired

Heat oil, zinc and beeswax in a microwave safe dish for approximately 25 seconds or use a double broiler to bring it to approximately 90 degrees.

Slowly pour the tea mixture into the oil mixture. Whip or use a blender to combine the ingredients.

While I do add herbs & oils that contain beneficial compounds, I typically do not add color or fragrance to any product designed for damaged skin because additives can cause the irritation to worsen. If you prefer something other than the natural color or scent, you can add your favorite colorant, essential oils, or herbs to the mixture.

Remember that everyone's skin reacts differently. You should test the products on a less sensitive area before using them. You should also remember that even natural products have side effects. The appendix gives the most common expected benefits and results of these ingredients. You should review these entries before trying any recipe.

Skin Smoothing Lotion

This lovely light lotion is great for year round care. The corn flour provides a silky texture to the lotion that leaves the skin feeling supple and smooth while the natural humectants qualities of the glycerin attract moisture to provide a softening quality.

3 tbsp.   Glycerin

3 tbsp.   Corn Flour (cornstarch powder)

¼ cup   Rose Water

¼ cup   Distilled Water

                   Emulsifier & Thickener as desired

Mix all of the ingredients in a microwave safe dish and heat for approximately 1 minute until the mixture just begins to boil. Stir the mixture every 20-25 seconds during heating. You may also heat the mixture to a light boil in a double broiler.

The product will have its own natural scent and color, but if you desire a specific color to suit your needs or an aromatherapy benefit you may add your favorite colorant or essential oils to the recipe. While I do add herbs & oils that contain beneficial compounds, I typically do not add color or fragrance to any product designed for damaged skin because additives can cause the irritation to worsen. If you prefer something other than the natural color or scent, you can add your favorite colorant, essential oils, or herbs to the mixture.

Pour the finished lotion into a clean container and seal it tightly. Allow the lotion to cool completely before use.

To use pump or pour a small amount into the palm of your hand and massage gently into the skin. This lotion is more gel like so you will need to use care until you learn to manage the application.

Remember that everyone's skin reacts differently. You should test the products on a less sensitive area before using them. You should also remember that even natural products have side effects. The appendix gives the most common expected benefits and results of these ingredients. You should review these entries before trying any recipe.

Toning Lotion

This is an effective lotion for the body. It infuses the skin with various toning and emollient components while helping to reduce irritants that may cause future outbreaks.

1 tbsp.	Crushed Fennel Seeds
¼ cup	Distilled Water

Bring the water to a light boil. Remove the water from the heat and pour it over the fennel seeds. Allow the mixture to soak overnight. Drain the seeds from the liquid and discard the seeds. The liquid will act as the base for your recipe.

2 tbsp.	Grated Beeswax
1 tbsp.	Aloe Vera Gel

Combine beeswax and aloe vera gel in a microwave safe dish and heat it for approximately 30 seconds or until the ingredients are melted. You can also use a double broiler until the mixture turns to a smooth liquid or reaches approximately 90 degrees Fahrenheit.

Remove the mixture from the heat and allow it to cool to approximately 70 degrees.

Add

1 tsp.	Vitamin E oil
1 tbsp.	Jojoba Oil

Stir the oils into the beeswax mixture.

2 tbsp.	Aluminum Sulfate
3 tbsp.	Witch Hazel
3 tbsp.	Orange Flower Water
	Emulsifier & Thickener as desired

Use only *USP Grade for Cosmetic Use* aluminum sulfates.

Use only plastic or ceramic pans and utensils since aluminum sulfate can react with metals.

Dissolve the aluminum sulfate in the witch hazel and orange flower water.

Slowly pour the liquid solution into the oil base stirring well.

The product will have its own natural scent and color, but if you desire a specific color to suit your needs or an aromatherapy benefit you may add your favorite colorant or essential oils to the recipe. While I do add herbs & oils that contain beneficial compounds, I typically do not add color or fragrance to any product designed for damaged skin because additives can cause the irritation to worsen.

Spoon the finished liquid into a clean container with a tight fitting lid. Allow the mixture to cool completely before use.

Massage the lotion in to the skin twice daily for the most beneficial results.

Remember that everyone's skin reacts differently. You should test the products on a less sensitive area before using them. You should also remember that even natural products have side effects. The appendix gives the most common expected benefits and results of these ingredients. You should review these entries before trying any recipe.

Lotion to Silkening Powder

Any lotion in the recipe book can be turned into a silkening powder. This is wonderful for helping to hydrate & moisturize the skin while minimizing oil build up throughout the day. As the lotion absorbs into the skin, the powder stays on the surface.

Start with any lotion base you prefer.

Add 2 tablespoons of cornstarch or another preferred powder to your lotion.

Whip the mixture until it is well blended.

Apply it your skin as you would any lotion.

As it dries, it leaves a beautiful silky feeling behind.

Scar Reduction Serum

Sometimes blemishes leave marks. When these marks are pigmentation scars, you can help to fade them with the proper treatments. This is one of my favorites and best of all it works on freckles too!

2 tsp.	Kukui Nut Oil
1 tsp.	Powdered Gotu Kola
½ tsp	Vitamin E Oil
½ tsp	Magnolia Oil
	Emulsifier & Thickener as desired

Blend all of the oils in a clean container with a tight fitting lid.

While I do add herbs & oils that contain beneficial compounds, I typically do not add color or fragrance to any product designed for damaged skin because additives can cause the irritation to worsen. If you prefer something other than the natural color or scent, you can add your favorite colorant, essential oils, or herbs to the mixture.

The oils may separate if they are allowed to sit. Shake the mixture well before each use. Dab the oils onto areas with dark pigmentation. Allow the oils to absorb naturally. Do not rinse the oils from your skin. The fading action is most pronounced when the oils are applied at least 3 times a day and not diluted with other lotions or make up.

Remember that everyone's skin reacts differently. You should test the products on a less sensitive area before using them. You should also remember that even natural products have side effects. The appendix gives the most common expected benefits and results of these ingredients. You should review these entries before trying any recipe.

Alternative Scar Reduction Gel

This gel is a nice alternative scar reducing cream. It works best as a nighttime treatment because the gel tends to be a little shiny when it dries. This may not be as powerful as the Scar Reduction Serum but it also tends to be less irritating.

2 tsp   Aloe Vera Gel

2 tsp   Asphodelus

Blend the ingredients in a clean container with a tight fitting lid.

While I do add herbs & oils that contain beneficial compounds, I typically do not add color or fragrance to any product designed for damaged skin because additives can cause the irritation to worsen. If you prefer something other than the natural color or scent, you can add your favorite colorant, essential oils, or herbs to the mixture.

Apply the lotion to the skin in a thin layer. Do not rinse the lotion from the skin.

Remember that everyone's skin reacts differently. You should test the products on a less sensitive area before using them. You should also remember that even natural products have side effects. The appendix gives the most common expected benefits and results of these ingredients. You should review these entries before trying any recipe.

CHAPTER 7

Mineral Makeup

Once your skin is clean, treated, and hydrated you may want to add makeup to enhance your overall appearance. Selecting a makeup can be a tough decision for those who suffer from acne outbreaks. You certainly do not want to select a makeup that is going to undo all that you have achieved through selective skin treatments. One solution that is becoming a popular choice among acne sufferers is mineral makeup.

Mineral make up has been used for hundreds, even thousands of years across the globe. Over the last few years, interest in this natural skin colorant has undergone a tremendous boost. Many companies have developed lines of mineral makeup. Each touts the benefits of their line over the next. Whether one is better than another is a matter of opinion and I am not going to express mine here!

What I am going to do is tell you a few of the benefits all of these lines (and homemade mineral makeup) offer to you. Then, I will show you the recipe that I use to make mineral make up at home for myself, my daughter, my daughter's classmates and friends and even some of my friends and family. I like the make up that I make at home, love that I can feel comfortable having 'girl's day' with my 9 year old and her friends without worrying that I am ruining their skin, and especially love that it costs me pennies to make a years supply of makeup for everyone!

Mineral makeup is a wholly natural make up product created mostly from powdered minerals. The benefits of mineral make up are numerous but the most influential factor to most people is that it is 100% natural.

BENEFITS:

- Mineral makeup is made from zinc and titanium dioxide so it is a natural sunscreen. Depending on how much you use SPF can range from 10 to 20.

- Mineral makeup is typically Distilled Water resistant. That is not to say Distilled Waterproof but it does last much better while swimming or during Distilled Water sports than many other make up products.

- Mineral makeup is long-lasting, bearing up better to long days, outdoor activity, and even naps than more traditional make up products.

- Mineral makeup contains ingredients that have special properties of their own. In addition to offering a natural sunscreen, you receive the side-benefits of each ingredient. If you look at the recipe for mineral base, you will see that zinc oxide is a main component. Zinc oxide has natural anti-inflammatory properties so the make up you make with zinc oxide will too!

- When applied correctly, the coverage offered by mineral make up is lightweight and complete. This makes it perfect for all skin types – from young to old, oily to dry and everything in between.

- Mineral make up is non-comedogenic and (unless you add oils to the recipe) oil free! This means it is less harmful and irritating to your skin. Some makers say it is so clean you can even sleep in it!

- Mineral make up is all-natural and the ingredients (unless you add oils to the recipe) do not go bad. That means you do not have to add any preservatives to the mix making it healthier and more natural than the next makeup!

- Mineral make up is fast and easy to apply.

- Mineral make up is VERY inexpensive to make at home.

Base or Foundation

Base or foundation is applied all over the face to create a smooth texture, even skin tone, and flawless finish.

4 tsp	Micronized Titanium Dioxide
1 ½ tsp	Bismuth Oxychloride
2 tsp	Zinc Oxide – Low Micron
½ tsp	Magnesium Stearate

Mix base ingredients by blending well. You can use a mortar / pestle, metal spoon and bowl, or food processor to blend the ingredients.

Slowly add the pigment colorant to the mix.

+/- to preference

¼ tsp	Yellow Iron Oxide
Pinch	Brown Iron Oxide
Pinch	Red Iron Oxide
½ tsp	Sericite Mica - matte or translucent finish to suit final goals

You can change the tint of the final product to suit your skin tone and color preferences.

For darker shades, add more of any of the iron oxides.

For lighter shades, add more titanium dioxide or some serecite mica.

Some people have reported that Bismuth Oxychloride causes irritation and redness. If you have sensitive skin or develop a reaction to the recipe, you may try using less or no Bismuth Oxychloride in your recipe.

Some people might want to experiment with different color additives to correct or address certain problems. You could start with:

Yellow Oxide   Brightens dull complexions and counteracts redness.

Chromium Oxide Green   Counters redness from seborrhea, acne, or irritated skin.

Ultramarine Violet Counters yellow or sallow skin tones; minimizes yellowish bruises.

Ultramarine Blue   Counters orange tones that may result from sunless tanning products.

LIQUID APPLICATION – some people prefer a bit more moisture in their makeup or like a liquid application more than a dry application. We make a liquid application by adding the powder mixture to our preferred moisturizer. The consistency of the liquid application is entirely a matter of preference. You will want to experiment by slowly adding the mineral mixture to your favorite moisturizer until you achieve the consistency and coverage amount you desire. The consistency ranges from full coverage matt to a lightweight tinted moisturizer.

Mineral Veil – Finish Powder

Mineral Veil is also called a finish powder and gives the face a translucent glow. It is applied on top of all other makeup.

3 tsp	Sericite Mica – Matte
1 tsp	Corn Starch
½ tsp	Boron Nitrate
½ tsp	Magnesium Stearate

Mix base ingredients by blending well. You can use a mortar / pestle, metal spoon and bowl, or food processor to blend the ingredients.

Slowly add the pigment colorant to the mix.

+/- to preference

Pinch	Yellow Iron Oxide
Pinch	Pink
Pinch	Brown Iron Oxide

You can change the tint of the final product to suit your skin tone and color preferences.

For darker shades, add more of any of the iron oxides.

For lighter shades, add more Corn Starch.

Concealer

A concealer is similar to a foundation in composition with a few simple modifications. Concealer tends to be a couple of shades lighter than your foundation, provides more coverage and is more matte in finish.

½ tbsp	Micronized Titanium Dioxide
½ tbsp	Serecite Mica – Matte
¼ tbsp	Magnesium Stearate

Mix base ingredients by blending well. You can use a mortar / pestle, metal spoon and bowl, or food processor to blend the ingredients.

Slowly add the pigment colorant to the mix.

+/- to preference

1/16 tbsp	Yellow Iron Oxide
Pinch	Light Red or Orange Iron Oxide

You can change the tint of the final product to suit your skin tone and color preferences.

For darker shades, add more of any of the iron oxides.

For lighter shades, add more titanium dioxide or some serecite mica.

Some people might want to experiment with different color additives to correct or address certain problems. You could start with:

Yellow Oxide Brightens dull complexions or counteracts redness.

Chromium Green Counters redness from seborrhea, acne, or irritated skin.

Ultramarine Violet Counters yellow or sallow skin tones; minimizes yellowish bruises.

Ultramarine Blue Counters orange tones that may result from sunless tanning products.

LIQUID APPLICATION - Some people prefer a bit more moisture in their makeup or like a liquid application more than a dry application. We make a liquid application by adding the powder mixture to our preferred moisturizer. The consistency of the liquid application is entirely a matter of preference. You will want to experiment by slowly adding the powder mixture to your favorite moisturizer until you achieve the consistency and coverage amount you desire.

Concealer often needs to be a bit heavier in weight. To create a heavier blend, you may want to try adding more mineral to the moisturizer or use a very heavy moisturizer as the base.

APPLICATION – DRY - To apply concealer in dry or powder form, first apply your foundation then use a small brush to apply the concealer directly to problem areas. Use a larger "Kabuki" brush to blend.

APPLICATION – WET - To apply concealer wet, put a small amount in the palm of your hand, add a small amount of Distilled Water or moisturizer as desired, and apply with a brush or a sponge to problem areas. By applying wet, you can target larger problem areas. Allow concealer to dry after application. Apply powdered foundation over the concealer to blend and finish.

Bronzer

A bronzer gives extra color where the sun hits the face. The sun leaves a bronze or rosy hue behind. The bronzer gives you the ability to infuse a fresh, healthy glow to your skin without the dangers of spending the day in the sun.

2 tsp   Micronized Titanium Dioxide

1/3 tsp   Magnesium Stearate

Mix base ingredients by blending well. You can use a mortar / pestle, metal spoon and bowl, or food processor to blend the ingredients.

Slowly add the pigment colorant to the mix.

+/- to preference

½ tsp   Yellow Iron Oxide

½ tsp   Brown Iron Oxide

½ tsp   Red Iron Oxide

1 tsp   Sericite Mica – pearl finish

½ tsp   Bronze mica

You can change the tint of the final product to suit your skin tone and color preferences.

For darker shades, add more of any of the iron oxides.

For lighter shades, add more titanium dioxide or serecite mica.

Eye Shadow

Eye Shadow is used to give extra attention to the eyes.

1 tbsp	Micronized Titanium Dioxide
½ tsp	Magnesium Stearate
1 tsp	Sericite Mica – Pearl or Matte as preferred

Pearl Sericite will give you a shimmer effect eye shadow

Matte Sericite will give you a low luster eye shadow

Mix base ingredients by blending well. You can use a mortar / pestle, metal spoon and bowl, or food processor to blend the ingredients.

Slowly add the pigment colorant to the mix.

+/- to preference

½ tsp   Iron Oxide color of your choice

Start with ½ tsp and increase until desired color is obtained

We enjoy mixing multiple colors to attain a shadow that is specific to us. If you custom mix your shadow to your personal preference – DO NOT forget to write down what you did so you can repeat it later.

You can change the tint of the final product to suit your skin tone and color preferences.

For darker shades, add more of any of the iron oxides.

For lighter shades, add more titanium dioxide or some serecite mica.

Blush

Blush is used to accent the cheekbones and provide a healthy color to the face.

2 ¾ tsp	Sericite Mica
1/4 tsp	Micronized Titanium Dioxide
1/16 tsp	Arrowroot Powder

Mix base ingredients by blending well. You can use a mortar / pestle, metal spoon and bowl, or food processor to blend the ingredients.

Slowly add the pigment colorant to the mix.

+/- to preference

| 1/16 tsp | Red Iron Oxide |

Start with 1/16 tsp and increase until desired color is obtained

We enjoy mixing multiple colors to attain a shadow that is specific to us. If you custom mix your shadow to your personal preference – DO NOT forget to write down what you did so you can repeat it later.

Appendix A
Acne Care
Ingredients

All natural make up and personal care products have become 'the thing' for many people. Whether from a desire to reduce chemical usage, reduce expenses, address specific issues better than the mass market products or just live a more natural life, more and more people I speak with are making their own cleaners, make-up and beauty products.

My family has used 'natural' products for years. My mother and grandmother both had skin and allergy issues and passed many home cleaning, personal care, and other product ideas down to my daughter and I. My daughter was born with the same sensitive skin and had the added issue of being a chemical reactive asthmatic.

I have posted many video and recipe instructions for the products that we use and enjoy the most. However, there are many reasons that people want to make their own natural products and your needs may not be the same as ours. There are also many combinations of product components that we have not yet tried. The following pages list some of the most commonly used elements and their supposed properties and effects.

Before you begin using the included ingredient lists, please remember that the properties and effects shown for each ingredient has not been fully proven and in many cases endorsed by the FDA or AMA. Whenever I am aware of a particular approval or endorsement, have included the information. All of this information has been gathered over years of use, chats with other people, and trial and error research. Please use your care and your own common sense when trying any of the included ingredients.

Enjoy!

Abscess Root
American Greek Valerian, Abscess Root, Blue Bells, False Jacob's ladder, Sweatroot

Botanical Name:
Polemonium reptans

Common Uses:
Acne

Traditional Uses:
Abscess Root is believed to be a beneficial wash for the treatment of certain types of acne and is traditionally used to cleanse and speed the healing of minor wounds.

Parts Used:
Root

Side Effects:
Abscess Root is not recommended for use by women who are pregnant or nursing.

Abscess Root may cause profuse sweating.

Additional uses and side effects may exist but further research is necessary to determine the exact properties and effects of the root.

General:
Abscess root is a perennial growing up to 1 foot by 1 foot native to Eastern North America and hardy to zone 4 that is easily propagated by seed in light sandy soil or medium loamy soil with good drainage

Abscess Root is harvested in the summer or fall, dried and powdered for use in traditional medicinal infusions up to 3 times daily and harvested after first frost for use in decoctions, tinctures, or inhalants up to 3 times daily. The most common traditional method is to make an alcohol tincture delivered as 1 ounce up to 3 times daily.

Abuta
Abuta, Batua, False Pareira, Patha, Velvetleaf

Botanical Name:
Cissampelos pareira

Common Uses:
Acne

Traditional Uses:
Abuta has been used as part of a traditional tea treatment to ease the number and severity of certain types of acne outbreaks.

Abuta is traditionally crushed and included in an alcohol poultice for relief from the pain and inflammation associated with arthritis, joint injury and rheumatism.

Parts Used:
Bark, Root

Side Effects:
Abuta is not recommended for use by women who are pregnant or nursing.

Abuta may affect estrogen levels and is not recommended for women who have an estrogen condition like endometriosis, fibroids or estrogen sensitive cancer.

Additional uses and side effects may exist but further research is necessary to determine the exact properties and effects.

General:
Abuta is a flowering plant propagated by seed and native to the rainforest. The root and bark are harvested, dried and powdered for use as an infusion or topical preparation.

Acacia - Gum
Acacia, Gum Arabic

Botanical Name:
Acacia senegal

Common Uses:
Binding Agents, Natural Skin Care

Traditional Uses:
Acacia Gum is often used as a stabilizer in creams and lotions and helps to improve the texture of semi-solid preparations.

Parts Used:
Gum

Side Effects:
Acacia is not recommended for use by women who are pregnant or nursing.

Acacia may cause an allergic reaction in some people.

Additional uses and side effects may exist but further research is necessary to determine the exact properties and effects of the root.

General:
Acacia is native to the semi-desert regions of Africa, Pakistan and India where the gum resin is

harvested for use as a thickening agent or added to foods, cosmetic, or medicinal preparations.

Acacia Gum powder is soluble in Distilled Water so it can be added to creams, lotions, liquid poultices, tooth care products, food products, and other items to stabilize the liquid and improve the texture of the final product.

1 tablespoon powdered gum to 3 tablespoons fluid creates a syrupy result.

Acacia Bark

Botanical Name:
Acacia decurrens

Common Uses:
Acne, Eczema, Natural Skin & Hair Care

Traditional Uses:
An herbal infusion of Acacia is believed to be a helpful component in anti-septic washes for the treatment of acne, eczema, and contact dermatitis.

Powdered Acacia is used as a binding agent for lotions, ointments and other semi-solids and is often used in natural skin care products.

Acacia bark is soluble in cold Distilled Water.

Powdered Acacia Bark is added as a component in lotions to tighten skin and may help heal irritation.

Parts Used:
Bark - Powdered

Side Effects:
Acacia is not recommended for use by women who are pregnant or nursing.

Some people may have an allergic reaction to Acacia.

Overuse of Acacia can cause indigestion or constipation in some people.

Additional uses and side effects may exist but further research is necessary to determine the exact properties and effects.

General:
Acacia is native to the semi-desert regions of Africa, Pakistan and India. Acacia bark contains high levels of tannins and it is frequently used for tanning hides or is dried, and powdered for use in topical, culinary, and medicinal preparations.

1 tablespoon powdered bark to 3 tablespoons fluid creates a syrupy result.

Acai Berry

Botanical Names:
Euterpe oleracea

Common Uses:
Natural Skin Care

Traditional Use:
Acai oil is full of antioxidants and is a prized component in natural skin care treatments geared toward anti-aging.

Part Used:
Berries, Juices, Oil

Side Effects:
Acai berry is not recommended for women who are pregnant or nursing.

Acai may cause an allergic reaction in some sensitive people.

Additional uses and side effects may exist but further research is necessary to determine the exact properties and effects.

General:
Acai Berry is native to Central and South America and produces a reddish purple berry that has become popular in weight loss and immunity boosting supplements. It is available in many natural supplement stores as a prepared supplement or freeze-dried powder.

Acai Berry is traditionally taken as a pill or food additive and is often used in weight reduction recipes like fruit smoothies & yogurt.

Acacia, Umbrella Thorn

Botanical Name:
Acacia tortilis

Common Uses:
Skin Irritation, Thickening Agent

Traditional Use:
Powdered Umbrella Thorn bark is traditionally sprinkled over minor wounds and abrasions to aid in removing surface bacteria while maximizing the bodies healing ability.

Umbrella Thorn gum is used as a thickening alternative to Gum Arabic in many preparations.

Parts Used:
Bark, Leaf, Seed – Gum

Side Effects:
Acacia Umbrella Thorn is not recommended for use by women who are pregnant or nursing.

Umbrella Thorn may have a mild sedative effect and you should not drive or operate heavy machinery while using Umbrella Thorn.

Umbrella Thorn is recommended for topical use only.

Additional uses and side effects may exist but further research is necessary to determine the exact properties and effects.

General:
Umbrella Thorn is a canopied tree native to Africa that can also be found growing in the Middle East where it is harvested, dried, and powdered for use as a food product or in traditional supplement applications.

Adder's Tongue
Adder's Tongue, Dog's Tooth, Fawn Lilly

Botanical Name:
Erythronium americanum

Common Uses:
Acne, Natural Skin Care, Skin Eruptions

Traditional Use:
Topical ointments made from the leaf and spikes of the Adder's Tongue are used in traditional washes for treating acne, wounds, eruptive skin irritations, and ulcers.

Fresh Adder's Tongue leaves are traditionally mixed into a lotion base or poultice to soothe bruised skin.

Adder's Tongue is emollient and the leaves are applied directly or in a lotion base to help smooth and soften the skin.

Part Used:
Bulbs, Leaves, Oils, Spike

Side Effects:
Adder's Tongue is not recommended for women who are pregnant or nursing.

People who are allergic to plants in the lily family may have an allergic reaction to this plant.

Additional uses and side effects may exist but further research is necessary to determine the exact properties and effects.

General:
Adder's Tongue is native to the United States where it can be found growing in open woodlands and cultivated gardens. The leaves are harvested for use in poultices and infusions. Adder's Tongue is most commonly used in the treatment of skin conditions including acne related eruptions, environmental reactions, and ulcers.

Aerva
Aerva, Astmabayata, Bameha, Bhadram, Chaya, Cherula

Botanical Name:
Aerva lanata

Common Uses:
Acne, Contact Dermatitis, Eczema, Skin Irritation

Traditional Use:
Powdered Aerva is traditionally included in poultices and washes to relieve minor skin irritation & inflammation as a treatment component for some types of acne, eczema, and contact dermatitis.

Part Used:
Leaves, Roots

Side Effects:
Areca is not recommended for use by women who are pregnant or nursing.

Areca may cause an allergic reaction in come people.

Additional uses and side effects may exist but further research is necessary to determine the exact properties and effects of use.

General:
Aerva is a woody succulent that grows wild in Africa and India and is cultivated elsewhere for use as a vegetable or as a medicinal. The flowers are sold in a commercial preparation in India.

Agar

Botanical Name:
Gelidium amansii

Common Uses:
Natural Hair & Skin Care

Traditional Use:
Agar is a gelatin like thickening agent that shows a good balance between thickening and melting points making it a frequently used ingredient in cooking and natural product recipes.

Part Used:
Whole

Side Effects:
Agar is not recommended for use by women who are pregnant or nursing.

Agar is not recommended for individuals who have bowel obstruction.

Agar may result in poor absorption of nutrients and other medicines.

Agar must be taken with plenty of Distilled Water.

If abdominal pain, chest pain, or difficulty swallowing occur you should see a physician or qualified herbalist immediately.

Additional uses and side effects may exist but further research is necessary to determine the exact properties and effects of use.

General:
Agar is a form of seaweed that is frequently used as a thickening agent in supplement, culinary, and cosmetic treatments. 1 teaspoon powder to 1 cup of boiling Distilled Water creates a jelly like substance suitable for inclusion in a variety of recipes or traditionally delivered as 1 ounce of the gel up to 3 times daily with an adequate amount of fluids to be taken in addition to the gel.

Agrimony
Agrimony, Church Steeples, Cocklebur, Stickwort

Botanical Name:
Agrimonia eupatoria

Common Uses:
Acne, Eczema, Skin Inflammation

Traditional Use:
Agrimony is traditionally used as a skin wash to help alleviate the inflammation and irritants that cause certain types of acne.

Agrimony is used in traditional wash or ointment preparations to improve chronic skin conditions like eczema and contact dermatitis.

Part Used:

Leaf, Stem - Oil

Side Effects:
Agrimony is not recommended for use by women who are pregnant or nursing.

Tannins have been linked to liver function toxicity in high levels.

Overuse of Agrimony may cause gastrointestinal upset and may aggravate constipation.

Agrimony may cause photosensitivity in some people.

Additional uses and side effects may exist but further research is necessary to determine the exact properties and effects of the root.

General:
Agrimony is a hardy perennial, flowering plant native to Asia, Europe, and North America. It grows 3-4 feet tall and blooms yellow flowers in July and August that have been used as a supplement since the time of the Ancient Greeks. Agrimony is harvested by cutting the plant a few inches above the ground and air-drying them for use as a traditional supplement tea or decoction up to 3 times daily. External washes, poultices, and treatments typically use powdered Agrimony or oils at a rate of 10% total volume.

Alder Buckthorn
Alder Buckthorn, Alder Dogwood, Arrow Wood, Black Dogwood, Frangula, Glossy Buckthorn

Botanical Name:
Rhamnus frangula

Common Uses:
Acne

Traditional Use:
Alder Buckthorn is traditionally used as part of a daily treatment to reduce acne eruptions.

Part Used:
Bark, Berry, Leaf

Side Effects:
Alder Buckthorn is not recommended for use by women who are pregnant or nursing

Alder Buckthorn is not recommended for use in children's treatments.

Alder Buckthorn is not recommended for use by people with Crohn's Disease, IBS, or Ulcerative Colitis.

Alder Buckthorn may cause cramps, diarrhea,
Distilled Water stools, or vomiting.

Alder Buckthorn berries are purgative and can be
dangerous if taken in excess.

Overuse of Alder Buckthorn may cause low
potassium, heart problems, muscle weakness, and
bleeding.

Additional uses and side effects may exist but
further research is necessary to determine the
exact properties and effects of use.

General:
Alder Buckthorn is native to Africa, Asia, and
Europe and has been naturalized to parts of North
America. It is used in a variety of manufacturing
items including gunpowder, fuses, nails, and
veneer. The bark, berry, and leaf are also
harvested in the fall, dried, and powdered for use
in traditional medicinal teas up to 3 times daily.

Almond Oil
Botanical Name:
Prunus communis

Common Uses:
Contact Dermatitis, Natural Skin & Hair Care, Skin
Irritation - Eczema, Carrier Oil

Traditional Use:
Almond oil is easily absorbed with natural
astringent & emollient actions making it useful in
natural hair & skin care products.

Almond oil is used as a traditional skin lotion
component to alleviate itchy skin conditions like
contact dermatitis.

Almond is used in lotions and ointments to alleviate
itchy skin conditions and promote a clear, younger
looking complexion in any skin type.

Part Used:
Nut – Flour, Milk, Oil

Side Effects:
Almond oil should be extracted from the almond
meat only.

Almond hull oils may be toxic in large quantities.

Additional uses and side effects may exist but
further research is necessary to determine the
exact properties and effects of use.

Aloe
Aloe, Aloe Vera, Burn Plant, Elephant's Gall, Lily of
the Desert

Botanical Name:
Aloe Vera, Aloe barbadensis

Common Uses:
Acne, Natural Skin & Hair Care, Skin Rash Treatment
– eczema, poison ivy, ringworm, psoriasis, Sun Burn
Relief

Traditional Use:
Aloe is soothing, anti-inflammatory, and
antibacterial making it a potentially beneficial
ingredient for the treatment of acne.

Aloe gel is often used as a burn relief ointment.
Most treatments thicken the juice with seaweed for
easier application.

Aloe is sometimes used to treat minor skin wounds
and abrasions. Aloe is believed speed wound
healing by improving blood circulation and
preventing cell death.

Aloe is emollient & believed to stimulate collagen
regeneration making it a beneficial ingredient in
natural skin and hair care products.

Aloe can be used in preparations to relieve the
itchiness of eczema, poison ivy, ringworm, and
psoriasis. It is typically created in an ointment using
.5% aloe to a base.

Aloe is traditionally used as a poultice for wound
care because it has antibacterial, antifungal, and
antiviral compounds that help to prevent wound
infections.

Part Used:
Gel, Juice, Leaf

Side Effects:
Aloe bitters and aloe juice should not be taken
internally during pregnancy or menstruation or in
cases of rectal bleeding.

The laxative compounds in aloe are passed into
mother's milk, so nursing mothers should avoid
internal use of aloe.

Aloe can cause intense intestinal cramps if
overused.

Overuse of aloe juice can cause diarrhea.

The FDA banned the use of aloe as a laxative
ingredient in over-the-counter drug products in
2002, but it is widely used outside the United States.

The oral consumption of aloe leaf may cause cancer.

Consumption of aloe may cause lowered glucose levels.

Additional uses and side effects may exist but further research is necessary to determine the exact properties and effects of use.

General:
Aloe is native to Africa but can be grown as a garden plant in other warm climates and is cultivated as an indoor plant worldwide. Aloe is related to the cactus and each part of the plant contains substances that are used in supplement treatments. The Aloe leaves contain a gel that is used as a topical ointment. The green part of the leaf that surrounds the gel is used to produce aloe juice or dried latex.

Aloe Butter is an extract of aloe in a coconut oil base. It is solid at room temperature but melts on the skin. It is traditionally incorporated into lotions & creams at a rate of 3-5%, in balms at a rate of 5-100%, and in conditioners at a rate of 2-5%.

Aloe Oil is used at a rate of 5-10% in recipes to add healing properties while lowering the risk of bacterial or mold growth.

Aloeswood
Agarwood, Aloeswood, Oudh

Botanical Name:
Aquilaria malaccensis

Common Uses:
Acne, Pigmentation, Skin Tonic

Traditional Use:
Aloeswood bark is traditionally used to help detoxify the body in the treatment of acne, gout, and rheumatism.

Aloeswood is traditionally used in skin tonic mixtures and may have pigment restoration qualities.

Powdered Aloeswood is traditionally sprinkled as an antiseptic on open wounds.

Part Used:
Wood, Bark – Powdered

Side Effects:
Additional uses and side effects may exist but further research is necessary to determine the exact properties and effects of use.

General:
Aloeswood comes from the Aquilaria Tree found growing naturally in Cambodia, India, and Vietnam and cultivated elsewhere. Aloeswood is commonly harvested, dried, and powdered for use as an incense, fabrication, and supplement products.

Alstonia
Alstonia, Bitterbark, Devil's Bit, Devil Tree, Dita Bark, Fever Bark, Fever Bush

Botanical Name:
Alstonia constricta

Common Uses:
Acne

Traditional Use:
Alstonia bark tea has been used as a traditional supplement to help reduce the symptoms of rheumatism, gout, and acne.

Part Used:
Bark – Powdered

Side Effects:
Alstonia is not recommended for use by women who are pregnant or nursing.

Alstonia may lower blood pressure.

Alstonia may worsen the symptoms of depression.

Alstonia may aggravate stomach ulcers.

Overuse of Alstonia may cause allergic reactions, eye problems, irritability, heart problems, kidney problems, psychosis, and death.

Additional uses and side effects may exist but further research is necessary to determine the exact properties and effects of use.

General:
Alstonia is an evergreen tree that is found in much of the world. The bark of the Alstonia Tree is harvested, dried, and powdered for use in traditional supplements. The powder is traditionally dispersed as 1 part powder to 1 ½-cup Distilled Water given at a dose of 1 fluid ounce.

American Elder
American Elder, Elderberry, Elder Flower, Sambucus, Sauco, Sweet Elder

Botanical Name:

Sambucus canadensis

Common Uses:
Acne, Contact Dermatitis, Eczema

Traditional Uses:
The flowers of the American Elder have been included in traditional tea washes to alleviate certain types of acne and reduce the inflammation and irritation associated with contact dermatitis and eczema.

Parts Used:
Fruit, Flower

Side Effects:
Elder is not recommended for use beyond dietetic by women who are pregnant or nursing.

Unripe Elder fruit, leaves, and young stems may be toxic.

Additional uses and side effects may exist but further research is necessary to determine the exact properties and effects of use.

General:
American Elder is native to the United States but is cultivated in other regions where the fruit is used as a culinary to make wine or jam, the inner leaves, and bark are used as a dye product and the berries and flowers are harvested for use in traditional supplements.

Apple Vinegar
Apple Vinegar, Apple Cider Vinegar, Wine Vinegar

Botanical Name:
Malus domestica

Common Uses:
Natural Skin & Hair Care

Traditional Use:
Apple Vinegar has been used as a traditional skin wash to help speed healing in skin sores, ulcers, and wounds and to help remove warts.

Part Used:
Bark, Flowers, Fruit

Side Effects:
Apple seeds are toxic and should be consumed with caution.

Apple Cider Vinegar is not recommended for use beyond dietetic by women who are pregnant or nursing.

Apple Cider Vinegar may lower blood sugar.

Overuse of Apple Cider Vinegar may lower potassium.

Apple Cider Vinegar should be diluted before use.

Additional uses and side effects may exist for apple cider vinegar and whole books are available defining the believed properties and effects of use.

General:
The wild crab apple tree is now considered more beneficial than modernly cultivated apple trees.

Apples and Apple Vinegar are believed to have numerous uses and benefits. Entire books have been devoted to the uses of vinegar. The uses included here are believed to be the most commonly effective. You may wish to investigate a book specific to the uses and benefits of vinegar.

Apricot
Botanical Name:
Prunus armeniaca

Common Uses:
Contact Dermatitis, Eczema, Natural Skin &Hair Care, Skin Inflammation & Irritation

Carrier Oil

Traditional Use:
A decoction of the Apricot Bark is believed to be soothing to inflamed and irritated skin and is traditionally used to treat eczema and contact dermatitis.

Apricot Kernel oil is easily absorbed by the hair and skin making it a popular ingredient in natural skin & hair care recipes designed to infuse moisture without leaving a greasy feeling.

Apricot Kernel Oil is especially useful in moisturizing & nourishing aged, damaged, and sensitive skin.

Part Used:
Bark, Fruit, Seed - Oil

Side Effects:
Apricot is not recommended for use beyond dietary by women who are pregnant or nursing.

Apricot is generally considered safe when consumed as a food.

Apricot Kernel Oil is for external use only. Internal use of Apricot Kernel Oil is toxic.

Apricot may affect blood sugar and the dried fruit affects it more strongly than the fresh.

Additional uses and side effects may exist but further research is necessary to determine the exact properties and effects of use.

General:
Apricot is used as a food product by people around the world but it is also harvested for inclusion as a supplement and skin care ingredient. The apricot kernel is the seed of the fruit and is used to produce oils used for supplement purposes while the fruit itself is used in both topical and internal preparations.

Argan Oil
Botanical Name:
Argania spinosa

Common Uses:
Acne, Anti-Aging, Eczema, Healant, Natural Skin & Hair Care, Psoriasis

Traditional Use:
Argan Oil is rich in squalene and vitamins and is used to replace lost moisture while healing & protecting the skin. Argan oil has been used in traditional preparations to sooth skin ailments like acne, eczema, and psoriasis.

Argan Oil is rich in squalene and vitamins and is believed to replace lost moisture while limiting the effects of free radicals giving it a traditional use in anti-aging, smoothing, and strengthening products for the skin, hair, & nails.

Part Used:
Seed Oil

Side Effects:
Additional uses and side effects may exist but further research is necessary to determine the exact properties and effects of use.

General:
Argan Oil comes for the kernels of the Argan Tree native to Morocco and cultivation is being attempted elsewhere. Argan trees have been heavily commercialized and the oil has become very rare and costly. It is often combined with olive oil in treatments.

Arnica
Arnica, Leopardsbane, Mountain Daisy, Mountain Tobacco, Wolfsbane

Botanical Name:

Arnica montana

Common Uses:
Acne, Eczema

Traditional Use:
A wash of Arnica may help to improve inflammatory skin conditions like eczema and acne. It is traditionally used at a rate of 4 oz of Arnica Tincture added to 1 gallon of Distilled Water. Soak and repeat as needed.

Arnica is traditionally used in poultices & creams applied to areas of pain with swelling at a rate of 1 tbsp Arnica tincture to 1 cup of Distilled Water or cream base. The cream is believed to be most effective if used immediately following the appearance of swelling or injury and applied no more than two times in a 24-hour period.

Arnica is traditionally used in topical preparations to reduce pain and speed healing in minor wounds and ulcers.

Part Used:
Flower – Tincture, Root

Side Effects:
Arnica is not recommended for use by women who are pregnant or nursing.

Repeated applications of Arnica can cause skin irritation.

Arnica flower is for external use.

Arnica may have an effect on the heart when taken internally.

Arnica may cause an allergic reaction in people sensitive to plants in the sunflower family.

Arnica should not be applied to broken skin as too much of the herb might be absorbed.

Internal use of Arnica flowers can cause diarrhea, vomiting, and nosebleeds.

Additional uses and side effects may exist but further research is necessary to determine the exact properties and effects of use.

General:
Arnica is a sunflower grown in many regions of the world and has been used as a supplement for centuries. The root and flower are harvested, dried, and powdered for use in topical applications.

Arrowhead Grass
Botanical Name:
Viola japonica

Common Uses:
Skin Conditions – Acne, Boils, Ulcers

Traditional Use:
Arrowhead Grass is traditionally used as a topical cream component to help reduce inflammation and detoxify the skin while reducing the minor pain of boils, ulcers, acne and other skin eruptions.

Part Used:
Whole

Side Effects:
Arrowhead Grass is not recommended for use by women who are pregnant or nursing.

Arrowhead Grass may cause an allergic reaction in some people.
Additional uses and side effects may exist but further research is necessary to determine the exact properties and effects of use.

General:
Arrowhead grass is native to North America and is considered an invasive weed by some. It reproduces easily by rhizomes and seed preferring shallow, stagnant Distilled Water for optimal growth. The whole plant is harvested for use fresh or dried and powdered for use in traditional supplement infusions.

Arrowroot
Arrowroot, Maranta Starch

Botanical Name:
Maranta arundinacea

Common Uses:
Natural Hair & Skin Care, Thickening Agent

Traditional Use:
Arrowroot is used to thicken food, natural cosmetics, and supplement ointments, poultices, and creams.

Arrowroot has been used as a moist poultice to help draw poisons from bites & stings.

Part Used:
Root - Powdered

Side Effects:
Additional uses and side effects may exist but further research is necessary to determine the exact properties and effects of use.

General:
Arrowroot is native to Africa, Asia and Central America but has been naturalized to many warm regions where it is harvested, dried and powdered for use as a thickening agent in foods and cosmetics or as a traditional supplement.

Ashwagandha
Ajagandha, Amangura, Asan, Asana, Ashwagandha, Asoda, Hayahvaya, Indian Ginseng, Winter Cherry

Botanical Name:
Withania somnifera

Common Uses:
Acne

Traditional Use:
Ashwagandha is traditionally used to help detoxify the body and regulate hormones and is a common treatment types of acne.

Ashwagandha contains naturally occurring steroidal elements that are believed to be beneficial in treating inflammation. It also has a naturally occurring substance that may aid in decreasing the ability of painful stimuli to reach the brain making it traditional additive to creams and relaxants designed to treat pain including fibromyalgia pain, low back pain, and sciatica.

Part Used:
Leaves, Root

Side Effects:
Ashwagandha is not recommended for use by women who are pregnant or nursing.

Ashwagandha is a sedative and you should avoid operating heavy machinery while taking Ashwagandha.

Ashwagandha may lower blood pressure.

Ashwagandha may irritate the gastrointestinal tract.

Ashwagandha is not recommended for use without the guidance of a physician or qualified herbalist by people with an autoimmune disease like multiple sclerosis, lupus, or another disorder.

Additional uses and side effects may exist but further research is necessary to determine the exact properties and effects of use.

General:

139

Ashwagandha powder is used in traditional supplement teas or blended at a rate of 5 grams given or applied two times daily in food, cream, or another base for all conditions.

Asphodelus
Botanical Name:
Asphodelus albus

Common Uses:
Natural Skin Care – Hyper-Pigmentation, Scarring

Traditional Use:
Asphodelus is used as part of a topical ointment or cream for fading freckles, age spots, scar tissue, and other undesirable skin pigmentation.

Part Used:
Tubers - Oil

Side Effects:
Additional uses and side effects may exist but further research is necessary to determine the exact properties and effects of use.

Asphodelus may cause skin irritation in some people.

General:
Asphodelus is a perennial native to Central and Southern Europe but is cultivated as an ornamental in other parts of the world. It is used in cheese making, ornamental gardens, and traditional supplements. The tubers are traditionally harvested in the spring, dried, and powdered for use in topical preparations.

Avens
Avens, Benedict's Herb, Bennet's Root, Benoite, Blessed Herb, Colewort, Geum, Herb Bennet

Botanical Name:
Geum urbanum

Common Uses:
Canker Sores, Hyper-Pigmentation,

Traditional Use:
Avens is traditionally used as a component in canker sore treatment sticks, ointments, and as a gargle for mouth sores.

Avens has been used as a wash to help to decrease the appearance of freckles, age spots and other hyper-pigmentation.

Part Used:
Flower, Leaf, Root, Stem

Side Effects:
Avens is not recommended for use by women who are pregnant or nursing.

Additional uses and side effects may exist but further research is necessary to determine the exact properties and effects of use.

General:
Avens is found in Asia, Europe, and North America where the root is harvested for use in external washes, poultices and traditional supplement teas or as a powder supplement.

Avocado
Alligator Pear, Avocado

Botanical Name:
Persea americana

Common Uses:
Dry & Damaged Skin, Eczema, Natural Skin and Hair Care, Psoriasis

Traditional Use:
Avocado and Avocado oil are rich in Vitamins B, E, and K making them a key ingredient in many deep moisture skin masks, deep skin treatments, and hair treatments. Avocado is especially beneficial for mature or damaged skin as it helps to hydrate and nourish regenerating skin cells. Avocado is not recommended for oily skin and is frequently used for its ability to screen harmful sun rays.

Avocado oil may help to reduce the symptoms of extremely dry skin, eczema, and psoriasis when ingested as part of a supplement diet or applied as a topical ointment.

Part Used:
Fruit, Oil, Seed

Side Effects:
Avocado is not recommended for use beyond dietary by women who are pregnant or nursing.

Avocado may cause an allergic reaction in some people.

Additional uses and side effects may exist but further research is necessary to determine the exact properties and effects of use.

General:
Avocados are native to subtropical regions and do not tolerate frost. If you cultivate avocado indoors, you must have multiple trees to promote cross-pollination. To start a sprout pierce a seed from a

ripe avocado 3 or 4 times and place it in a glass of Distilled Water. Avocado is used as a food in many cultures and is a good source of potassium and Vitamin D. Avocado is also harvested for use in traditional supplements and dietary treatments.

Bakula

Botanical Name:
Mimusops elengi

Common Uses:
Acne

Traditional Use:
Bakula bark is traditionally included in washes or ointments to reduce the number and severity of certain types of acne outbreaks.

The bark is traditionally used in topical skin washes to help speed healing in wounds, ulcers, and eruptive skin conditions.

Part Used:
Bark, Flower, Fruit, Seed

Side Effects:
Additional uses and side effects may exist but further research is necessary to determine the exact properties and effects of use.

General:
Bakula is an evergreen tree native to Asia, Australia, Europe, and India where it has been used in traditional supplement treatments for centuries. It is harvested for its timber, fruit and supplement uses.

Balloon Vine
Botanical Name:
Cardiospermum halicacabum

Common Uses:
Acne, Contact Dermatitis, Eczema

Traditional Use:
Dried Balloon Vine leaves are traditionally boiled into a tea at a rate of 2 tablespoons to 1-cup Distilled Water that is used internally to reduce acne, eczema, and other skin conditions.

A poultice of balloon vine leaves can be applied as a hot poultice for relief from the pain and swelling associated with arthritis, joint injury, muscle pain and other painful inflammatory conditions.

Balloon Vine leaves have been used in traditional topical ointments to help alleviate the pain &

inflammation and speed healing in wounds and ulcers.

Part Used:
Leaves, Seeds, Vine - Whole

Side Effects:
Balloon Vine is not recommended for use by women who are pregnant or nursing.

Additional uses and side effects may exist but further research is necessary to determine the exact properties and effects of use.

General:
Balloon Vine is a perennial native to Central and South America and cultivated by seed as a climbing vine where it is harvested for use fresh or dried in traditional supplement preparations.

Basil
Albahaca, Basil, Garden Basil, Munjariki, Surasa, Varvara

Botanical Name:
Ocimum basilicum

Common Uses:
Acne, Natural Hair & Skin Care

Traditional Use:
Basil is traditionally included in skin washes to tone and brighten the skin and may be beneficial in treating certain types of bacterial acne.

Side Effects:
Basil is not recommended for use beyond dietary by women who are pregnant or nursing

Basil is not recommended for use beyond dietary in children's treatment.

Basil is not for long-term use.

Additional uses and side effects may exist but further research is necessary to determine the exact properties and effects of use.

General:
Basil is a commonly cultivated spice herb that grows easily from seed, Basil prefers full sunlight, fertile soil, and steady moisture and is often used as a seasoning or dried for use as a supplement tea.

Bay
Bay, Bay Laurel, Daphne, Grecian Laurel, Mediterranean Bay, Roman Laurel, Sweet Bay, True Bay

Botanical Name:
Laurus nobilis

Common Uses:
Natural Skin Care

Traditional Use:
Bay leaves added to a pot of boiling Distilled Water for use as a deep cleansing steam treatment for the face.

Part Used:
Fruit, Leaves, Oil

Side Effects:
Bay is not recommended for use beyond dietary by women who are pregnant or nursing.

Bay may cause an allergic reaction in some people.

Bay may irritate the skin and mucus membranes of some individuals and should be used with caution

Bay oil should not be taken internally. Oil is for external use only.

Additional uses and side effects may exist but further research is necessary to determine the exact properties and effects of use.

General:
Bay Laurel is not a winter hardy plant and should be brought indoors in much of the northern parts of the country. Bay prefers full sun light and good drainage.

Bayberry
Bayberry, Candleberry, Southern Bayberry, Tallow Shrub, Tung, Wax Myrtle, Waxberry

Botanical Name:
Myrica cerifera

Common Uses:
Acne

Traditional Use:
Bayberry contains natural antibacterial, anti-inflammatory, and astringent properties making it a potentially beneficial ingredient in the treatment of certain kinds of acne.

Part Used:
Bark, Berries, Roots

Side Effects:

Bayberry is not recommended for use by women who are pregnant or nursing.

Bayberry may elevate blood pressure.

Bayberry may deplete the body's natural potassium.

Bayberry may cause liver damage, nausea and vomiting.

Additional uses and side effects may exist but further research is necessary to determine the exact properties and effects of use.

General:
Bayberry grows in the United States and is known as Wax Myrtle in southern regions. Bayberry is often used as an ornamental shrub valued for its fragrant leaves and clusters of round berry like fruit. Bayberry can grow up to 6 feet in height in the North while the Wax Myrtle has been known to reach 40 feet in height in the South. The berries are often eaten as a food and the bark, berries, and root are harvested, dried, and powdered for use in traditional supplement preparations.

Bayberry – Sweet Gale
Bayberry, Bog Myrtle, Dutch Myrtle, Sweet Gale

Botanical Name:
Myrica gale

Common Uses:
Acne, Natural Skin Care – Redness, Seborrhea

Traditional Use:
Sweet Gale has been used in traditional topical washes and spot ointments to alleviate the severity of acne outbreaks and some types of skin redness including seborrhea.

Sweet Gale is used in natural skin care preparations to help reduce acne, inflammation redness, and seborrhea.

Part Used:
Branch, Leaf, Wax

Side Effects:
Sweet Gale is not recommended for use by women who are pregnant or nursing.

Sweet Gale has been used as an abortifacient in some cultures.

Additional uses and side effects may exist but further research is necessary to determine the exact properties and effects of use.

General:
Sweet Gale is a deciduous shrub native to Europe and North America where it is cultivated as an ornamental or harvested for use in topical preparations and as a flavoring.

Bergamot
Beebalm, Bergamot, Fragrant Balm, High Balm, Indian Plume, Mountain Balm

Botanical Name:
Bergamot didyma, Citrus bergamia

Common Uses:
Acne

Traditional Use:
Bergamot is an antibacterial, antiviral, analgesic and may be beneficial in treatments for certain types of acne when added to topical preparations at a rate of 1 to 10.

Part Used:
Fruit, Leaf, Peel Oil

Side Effects:
Bergamot is not recommended for use by women who are pregnant or nursing.

Bergamot is not recommended for use in children's treatments.

Bergamot increases sun sensitivity. Do not use on the skin when sun exposure is likely.

Additional uses and side effects may exist but further research is necessary to determine the exact properties and effects of use.

General:
Bergamot is native to Asia and can grow up to 16 feet in height. Bergamot is harvested for use in topical & internal preparations as well as in fragrances, inhalant therapy, and natural care products.

Birch Bark
Birch Bark, Cherry Birch, White Birch

Botanical Name:
Betula alba

Common Uses:
Acne, Eczema, Psoriasis

Traditional Use:

Birch Bark is traditionally incorporated into facial washes, lotions, & ointments designed to treat acne, eczema, psoriasis, and other skin disorders.

Birch has been used in skin washes to help disinfect wounds and promote healing.

Part Used:
Bark, Leaf, Root

Side Effects:
Birch may have a blood thinning action.

Birch is not recommended for use by women who are pregnant or nursing.

Birch is not recommended for use in children's treatments.

Birch is not recommended for use by individuals who are allergic to aspirin.

Birch oil is for external use only.

Additional uses and side effects may exist but further research is necessary to determine the exact properties and effects of use.

General:
Birch is native to cold, northern climates and is a deciduous tree that grows well in many types of soil and sun conditions. The bark and leaves are harvested, dried, and powdered for use in traditional supplement preparations and the oil is extracted from the leaf buds through steam distillation.

Silver Birch Betula pendula and Sweet Birch Betula lenta have been used in much the same way as the White Birch.

Bitter Dock
Bitter Dock, Broad Leaved Dock, Dock Leaf, Kettle Dock, Round Leaved Dock

Botanical Name:
Rumex obtusifolius

Common Uses:
Acne, Skin Eruptions

Traditional Use:
Bitter Dock has been used in traditional supplement washes to help alleviate acne and other eruptive skin conditions like chicken pox and contact dermatitis.

Bitter Dock tea has traditionally been used to detoxify the body and alleviate certain types of acne eruptions.

Part Used:
Leaf, Root

Side Effects:
Bitter Dock is not recommended for use by women who are pregnant, nursing, or trying to become pregnant.

Bitter Dock may cause an allergic reaction or skin irritation in some people.

Additional uses and side effects may exist but further research is necessary to determine the exact properties and effects of use.

General:
Bitter Dock is native to Europe and naturalized in much of North America. It grows deep taproots that are difficult to remove once established. It is considered an invasive weed by some growing well in all types of soil, Distilled Water, and sun conditions and resistant to cutting or trampling but it does provide nutritive feed for grazing animals. It is also harvested, dried, & powdered for use in traditional supplements.

Bitter Damson
Bitter Damson, Dysentery Bark, Mountain Damson, Simarouba, Slave Wood, Stave Wood

Botanical Name:
Simarouba amara

Common Uses:
Hyper-Pigmentation, Natural Skin Care

Traditional Uses:
Bitter Damson has been used in commercial and traditional topical preparations to fade freckles, age spots, and scarring and is valued as a natural skin care ingredient for its hydrating effect.

Parts Used:
Bark

Side Effects:
Bitter Damson is not for use by women who are pregnant or nursing.

Bitter Damson has been used as an abortifacient. Overuse of Bitter Damson may cause gastrointestinal upset.

Additional uses and side effects may exist but further research is necessary to determine the exact properties and effects of use.

General:
Bitter Damson is native to the Caribbean and South America where the bark is harvested, dried, and powdered for use in traditional supplement. Bitter Damson has recently gained interest by researches for its potential in treating viral infections, stimulating the immune system, and preventing or treating cancer.

Black Catechu
Black Catechu, Black Cutch, Cachou, Cutch, Gambier

Botanical Name:
Acacia catechu

Common Uses:
Acne, Contact Dermatitis, Eczema

Traditional Use:
Black Catechu has traditionally been incorporated into a wash for the treatment of acne, eczema, and other eruptive skin conditions.

Part Used:
Bark, Heartwood, Leaf

Side Effects:
Black Catchu is not recommended for use by women who are pregnant or nursing.

Black Catechu may lower blood pressure.

Additional uses and side effects may exist but further research is necessary to determine the exact properties and effects of use.

General:
Black Catechu is native to India where the bark is boiled to extract the dye properties or harvested, dried and powdered for use as a breath freshener, diuretic, colorant or traditional supplement.

Black Currant
Black Currant, Cassis

Botanical Name:
Ribes nigrum

Common Uses:
Natural Skin Care

Traditional Uses:

Blackcurrant oil is sometimes used as a replacement for evening primrose oil in natural skin care recipes.

Black Current has been used as a traditional wash to help speed the healing of minor wounds and skin ulcers.

Parts Used:
Fruit, Leaf, Seed – Oil

Side Effects:
Black Currant is not recommended for use by women who are pregnant or nursing.

Black current might slow blood clotting.

Additional uses and side effects may exist but further research is necessary to determine the exact properties and effects of use.

General:
Black Current is a berry native to Asia, Europe and cultivated elsewhere. The fruit is harvested as a food or drink component and for use as a dietary supplement. The leaves are harvested for use fresh or dried in traditional topical and tea supplements.

Black Jujube
Azufaifo, Badar, Ber, Black Date, Black Jujube, Chinese Date, Da Zao, Jujube Plum, Red Date

Botanical Name:
Ziziphus jujuba

Common Uses:
Natural Skin Care

Traditional Uses:
Jujube extracts are used in commercial and natural products to help reduce redness in the skin while combating wrinkles and premature aging.

Parts Used:
Fruit

Side Effects:
Jujube is not recommended for use by women who are pregnant or nursing.

Jujube is not recommended for use by people who are trying to conceive.

Jujube may lower the blood pressure.

Additional uses and side effects may exist but further research is necessary to determine the exact properties and effects of use.

General:
Black Jujube is a shrub or tree native to Asia and Europe. The fruit is harvested for use as a food product and for use in traditional supplements.

Black Seed
Ajenuz, Aranul, Baraka, Black Caraway, Black Seed, Chamuska, Fennel Flower, Fitch, Kalajaji, Mugrela, Nutmeg Flower, Upakuncika

Botanical Name:
Nigella sativa

Common Uses:
Acne

Traditional Use:
Black seed is used in traditional washes, ointments, or masks to help alleviate certain types of acne.

Part Used:
Oil, Seed

Side Effects:
Black Seed is not recommended for use by women who are pregnant or nursing.

Black Seed may act as a contraceptive and is not recommended for use by women who are trying to conceive.

Excessive use of Black Seed may cause skin irritation.

Additional uses and side effects may exist but further research is necessary to determine the exact properties and effects of use.

General:
Black Seeds are native to the Middle East and Western Asia. They are harvested, crushed and incorporated into a traditional supplement tea, added as a seasoning during cooking, or taken with a tincture base.

Blackthorn
Black Thorn, Blackthorn, Sloe, Wild Plum

Botanical Name:
Prunus spinosa

Common Uses:
Acne, Skin Inflammation

Traditional Uses:
Blackthorn flowers have been used in traditional topical preparations to deep cleanse the skin and alleviate certain types of acne.

Blackthorn flower is traditionally added to a poultice or wash to help sooth inflamed and irritated skin.

Parts Used:
Berry, Flower

Side Effects:
Black Thorn is not recommended for use by women who are pregnant or nursing.

Black Thorn may cause an allergic reaction in some people.

Additional uses and side effects may exist but further research is necessary to determine the exact properties and effects of use.

General:
Black Thorn is a deciduous shrub native to Africa, Asia, Europe and North America where it is cultivated as a naturally barbed hedge. The fruit is harvested as a jam or wine component and the fruit, flowers, and leaves are used in traditional supplements.

Blue Flag
Blue Flag, Dragon Flower, Flag Lily, Liver Lily, Wild Iris

Botanical Name:
Iris versicolor

Common Uses:
Acne, Eczema, Psoriasis

Traditional Use:
Blue Flag has been used as a traditional supplement to help detoxify the body and alleviate the severity of acne, eczema, and psoriasis outbreaks.

Part Used:
Rhizome – Root

Side Effects:
Blue Flag is not recommended for use by women who are pregnant or nursing.

The fresh root of the blue flag may cause intestinal upset, nausea, and vomiting. The dried root has a milder effect.

Additional uses and side effects may exist but further research is necessary to determine the exact properties and effects of use.

General:

Blue Flag is native to the marshes of the United States where the Native Americans harvested the rhizome, dried and powdered it for use in internal and external traditional supplements.

Boneset
Agueweed, Boneset, Crosswort, Feverwort, Indian Sage, Sweating Plant, Teasel, Thoroughwort, Wood Boneset

Botanical Name:
Eupatorium perfoliatum

Common Uses:
Acne, Contact Dermatitis, Eczema

Traditional Use:
Boneset has been used in traditional topical preparations to alleviate the symptoms of acne, eczema, and contact dermatitis.

Part Used:
Whole – After Flowering

Side Effects:
Boneset is not recommended for use by women who are pregnant or nursing.

Boneset is an immuno-stimulant and is not recommended for use by people who have an immune sensitive disorder like Multiple Sclerosis or Lupus.

Boneset may cause allergic reactions in those who suffer from seasonal allergies related to chamomile, ragwort, and others.

Overdose of Boneset may cause diarrhea, nausea, and vomiting.

Additional uses and side effects may exist but further research is necessary to determine the exact properties and effects of use.

General:
Boneset is native to the United States where it can be found growing wild in moist areas like swamp edges and stream banks. The entire herb is harvested after flowering and made into a traditional supplement tea up to 3 times daily or tincture traditionally given as ¾ teaspoon before meals.

Brown Kelp
Alginate, Brown Kelp, Pacific Kelp, Sea Kelp, Sea Whistle

Botanical Name:

Macrocystis pyrifera

Common Uses:
Natural Hair & Skin Care

Traditional Use:
Brown Kelp is used as a binding agent in supplement and natural care products and is sometimes used as a peel off facial masks.

Part Used:
Whole

Side Effects:
Brown kelp is not recommended for use by women who are pregnant or nursing.

Brown kelp is a source of iodine and should not be used by those who have hyperthyroidism.

Additional uses and side effects may exist but further research is necessary to determine the exact properties and effects of use.

General:
Brown kelp is found primarily along the California coastline and is harvested for use as a binding agent and in traditional supplements.

Buchu
Bookoo, Bucco, Buchu, Diosma

Botanical Name:
Agathosma betulina

Common Uses:
Acne

Traditional Use:
Buchu has been used in traditional supplements to help remove impurities and reduce the number and severity of flare ups in conditions like gout, rheumatism and certain types of acne.

Part Used:
Flowers, Leaves

Side Effects:
Buchu is not recommended for use beyond dietary by women who are pregnant or nursing.

Buchu is not recommended for use by people with kidney disease or a urinary tract infection.

The diuretic action of buchu reduces potassium levels in the blood.

Buchu is not for use by those with kidney disease.

Additional uses and side effects may exist but further research is necessary to determine the exact properties and effects of use.

General:
Buchu is native to wet areas of South Africa but can be grown indoors throughout the world. The oils are used in commercial and traditional supplements and the leaves are harvested and dried for use in traditional infusions.

Burdock
Arctium, Bardana, Bardane, Begger's Buttons, Burdock Root, Bur Oil, Burr Seed, Clotbur, Cocklebur, Gobo, Happy Major, Hardock, Harebur, Lappa, Love Leaves, Thorny Bur

Botanical Name:
Arctium lappa

Common Uses:
Acne

Traditional Use:
Burdock leaves, roots and seeds are believed to help to destroy certain bacteria and help to detoxify the body making them a traditional ingredient in the treatment of certain types of acne.

Part Used:
Leaf, Root, Seed

Side Effects:
Burdock is not recommended for use by women who are pregnant or nursing.

Burdock may cause an allergic reaction in some people.

Burdock may lower blood sugar.

Additional uses and side effects may exist but further research is necessary to determine the exact properties and effects of use.

General:
Burdock is native to Europe and Asia but has been introduced to North America and can often be found growing wild along ditches and roads. You can cultivate burdock from seeds directly in the garden or indoors. The roots are harvested in the first year for use as a food or made into traditional and commercial pharmaceuticals that are usually boiled at a rate of ½ - 1 teaspoon in 1 cup of Distilled Water, allowed to steep for 30 minutes. Up to 3 x's daily.

Butterbur
Blatterdock, Bog Rhubarb, Bogshorns, Butterbur, Butterfly Dock, Capdockin, Exwort, Flapperdock, Grand Bonnet, Langwort, Plague Root, Purple Butterbur, Umbrella Leaves

Botanical Name:
Petasites officinalis, Petasites hybridus

Common Uses:
Acne

Traditional Uses:
Fresh Butterbur leaves have been used as a topical treatment to alleviate the severity of acne outbreaks.

Parts Used:
Leaf

Side Effects:
Butterbur is not recommended for use by women who are pregnant or nursing.

Butterbur may cause an allergic reaction in some people.

Pyrrolizidine Alkaloid in Butterbur may cause worsen asthma symptoms in some people.

Butterbur may cause diarrhea, drowsiness, eye irritation, fatigue, headache, and upset stomach in some people.

Butterbur preparations may contain Pyrrolizidine Alkaloids and overuse can cause liver, lung, and circulatory system damage.

Additional uses and side effects may exist but further research is necessary to determine the exact properties and effects of use.

General:
Butterbur is native to Asia, Europe, and has been naturalized in North America where it can be found growing wild in wetlands or cultivated for use in traditional supplements. The bulb, leaf, and root are traditionally harvested for use in commercial and traditional preparations.

Caje Oil
Caje Oil, Huile, Niauli

Botanical Name:
Melaleuca viridiflora

Common Uses:
Acne, Skin Inflammation

Concentration, Focus

Traditional Uses:
Caje Oil has been used in traditional topical preparations to clean oily skin and combat bacteria in certain types of acne and to prevent infection and speed healing in skin ulcers and wounds.

Caje oil is applied directly to the throat, mouth, or skin to reduce inflammation and is traditionally believed to be most effective at treating bacterial infections and associated inflammation.

Parts Used:
Leaf, Twigs - Oil

Side Effects:
Caje Oil is not recommended for use by women who are pregnant or nursing.

Caje Oil is not recommended for use in children's treatments.

Caje Oil may cause diarrhea, nausea or vomiting.

Overuse of Caje Oil may cause breathing problems, circulation problems, and low blood pressure.

Additional uses and side effects may exist but further research is necessary to determine the exact properties and effects of use.

General:
Caje Oil is extracted from the leaves of the Melaleuca viridiflora plant and should not be confused with cajuput oil that is taken from a different species of the Melaleuca plant. The Melaleuca viridiflora is native to Australia where the bark is used as bedding, containers, and building shelter. The essential oil is extracted from young leaves and twigs for use in traditional supplement and disinfectant preparations.

Cajuput
Cajuput, Paperbark Tree, Swamp Tea Tree, White Tea Tree

Botanical Name:
Melaleuca leucadendron

Common Uses:
Acne, Eczema, Psoriasis

Traditional Use:
Cajuput oil has been used as part of a topical wash or ointment preparation to help alleviate the severity of acne, eczema and psoriasis outbreaks.

Part Used:
Leaves, Twigs

Side Effects:
Cajuput is not recommended for use by women who are pregnant or nursing.

Cajuput is not recommended in children's treatments.

Cajuput is not recommended for use by people with kidney problems.

Cajuput may worsen asthma symptoms in some people.

Cajuput may cause skin irritation. You should dilute it before applying cajuput to the skin and it is not recommended for use in the facial area.

Additional uses and side effects may exist but further research is necessary to determine the exact properties and effects of use.

General:
Cajuput is native to Australia and Asia preferring extremely wet conditions for optimal growth. Cajuput oil is extracted from the leaves and twigs of the tree and blended with other oils for use as a traditional supplement diluted at 5 drops cajuput to 1 tablespoon carrier oil.

Calendula
Bull Flower, Calendula, Gold Bloom, Holligold, Marigold, Mercadela, Pot Marigold, Zergul

Botanical Name:
Calendula officinalis

Common Uses:
Acne, Natural Skin Care

Traditional Use:
Calendula blossoms are anti-inflammatory, astringent, and anti-bacterial making them a traditional component in topical ointments for acne, burns, bruises, and minor wounds. Simmer with preferred ingredients and apply directly to the skin or include in a lotion recipe.

Calendula is traditionally used to cleanse and accelerate healing in minor wounds, bed sores, and ulcers.

Part Used:
Flowers, Oil

Side Effects:

Calendula is not recommended for use by women who are pregnant or nursing.

Calendula has been used as a male contraceptive and should not be used by men and women who are trying to conceive.

Calendula may cause an allergic reaction in some people.

Additional uses and side effects may exist but further research is necessary to determine the exact properties and effects of use.

General:
Calendula is native to the Mediterranean but is cultivated as an annual garden plant in much of the world. It is easy to grow from seed and should be harvested while in bloom. Calendula is traditionally dried and powdered for use as a tea up to 3 times daily but has also been used as a tincture or topical salve additive.

Camphor

Botanical Name:
Cinnamomum camphora

Common Uses:
Acne, Contact Dermatitis, Eczema, Natural Hair & Skin Care, Skin Irritation

Traditional Use:
Camphor oil is traditionally used in topical preparations to combat oily skin and acne.

Camphor has been approved for use in Europe as a topical cream to reduce skin itching and irritation from contact dermatitis, excessive dryness, and for conditions like eczema.

Part Used:
Wood – Steam Distilled Oils

Side Effects:
Camphor is not recommended for use by women who are pregnant or nursing.

Camphor is not recommended for topical applications in children.

Camphor may irritate skin and should not be applied to broken skin or large areas.

Use only cosmetic grade white camphor.

Camphor is for external use only.

Additional uses and side effects may exist but further research is necessary to determine the exact properties and effects of use.

General:
True Cinnamomum camphora is the waxy white substance extracted from the Camphor Laurel Tree native to Asia but camphor can be found in the bark of a variety of trees in smaller amounts than the Cinnamomum camphora. The bark is harvested and the oils extracted for use at a rate of up to 10% in traditional supplement preparations.

Carline Thistle
Carlina, Carline Thistle, Dwarf Carline, Ground Thistle, Stemless Carline

Botanical Name:
Carlina acaulis

Common Uses:
Acne, Contact Dermatitis, Eczema

Traditional Use:
Carline Thistle oils are traditionally included in a skin wash to alleviate the symptoms of acne, contact dermatitis, eczema, and skin ulcers and are believed to speed the healing process.

Carline Thistle is traditionally included in topical washes and ointments to prevent infection and speed healing of skin sores, ulcers and wounds.

Part Used:
Root - Oil

Side Effects:
Carline Thistle is not recommended for use by women who are pregnant or nursing.

Carline Thistle may cause an allergic reaction in some people.

Additional uses and side effects may exist but further research is necessary to determine the exact properties and effects of use.

General:
Carline Thistle is found in many areas of Europe and the United States where the root is harvested in the fall and dried for use in tea traditionally given at a rate of 2 teaspoons root powder to 1 cup of Distilled Water 3 times daily or steam distilled to extract the essential oils.

Carob

Algarrobo, Carob, Garrofero, Locust Bean, St. John's Bread, Sugar Pods

Botanical Name:
Ceratonia siliqua

Common Uses:
Natural Skin Care

Traditional Use:
Carob is included in natural skin care products to help to cleanse the face and tone the skin.

Part Used:
Bark, Seed

Side Effects:
Carob is not recommended for use beyond dietary by women who are pregnant or nursing.

Do not take Vitamin A supplements when using carob supplements.

Carob may increase the effects of digoxin in some individuals.

Additional uses and side effects may exist but further research is necessary to determine the exact properties and effects of use.

General:
Carob is native to Asia, Europe and the Mediterranean but it has been cultivated in North America. Carob is often used as a dietary additive by dissolving the powder in an equal part of cold liquid. Boil for 1 minute to create a thickening agent.

Carrot
Beesnest Plant, Bird's Nest Root, Carrot, Wild Carrot, Queen Anne's Lace

Botanical Name:
Daucus carota

Common Uses:
Natural Skin Care

Traditional Use:
Carrot seed oil helps to balance the oils in the skin, heal damage, and may be beneficial in aged skin care.

Part Used:
Leaf, Seed

Side Effects:
Carrot is not recommended for use by women who are pregnant or nursing.

Carrot Seed is a natural abortifacient.

Carrot Seed had been used as a morning after contraceptive in some cultures and is not recommended for use by women trying to conceive.

Wild Carrot may cause an allergic reaction in some people.

Wild Carrot may affect the kidneys.

Additional uses and side effects may exist but further research is necessary to determine the exact properties and effects of use.

General:
Wild carrot is native to Eastern North America, Europe, and Asia. It is often found growing in untended fields and along roadsides where it is harvested and juiced or made into a traditional supplement syrup.

Cedar - Atlantic
Atlantic Cedarwood, Atlas Cedarwood, Cedar

Botanical Name:
Cedurs atlantica

Common Uses:
Acne

Traditional Use:
Atlas cedar oil is an astringent, antiseptic that is often included in a skin wash for the treatment of acne, eczema, and other skin irritations.

Part Used:
Wood Oil

Side Effects:
Cedar is not recommended for use by women who are pregnant or nursing.

Cedar can cause skin irritation.

Additional uses and side effects may exist but further research is necessary to determine the exact properties and effects of use.

General:
Atlas Cedar is used more frequently in aromatherapy and is native to Morocco red cedar is native to North America.

Centaury
Bitter Herb, Centaury, Feverwort

Botanical Name:
Centaurium erythraea

Common Uses:
Hyper-Pigmentation, Natural Skin Care

Traditional Use:
An infusion of Centaury may help to clear blemishes, soften the skin and remove dark pigmentation so it is often used in natural skin care.

Part Used:
Flower, Leaf

Side Effects:
Centaury is not recommended for use by women who are pregnant or nursing.

Centaury should not be used with stomach or intestinal ulcers.

Additional uses and side effects may exist but further research is necessary to determine the exact properties and effects of use.

General:
Centaury is native to Asia, Africa and Europe and cultivated in the United States where it is harvested during the flowering season and dried quickly for use as a traditional tea supplement.

Chamomile - German
Blue Chamomile, German Chamomile, Hungarian Chamomile, Kamillen, Kleine Kamille, Manzanilla, Matricaire Camomille, Pin Heads, Sweet False Chamomile, True Chamomile, Wild Chamomile

Botanical Name:
Chamomilla recutita, Matricaria recutita

Common Uses:
Eczema, Natural Face, Hair & Skin Care

Traditional Use:
A poultice of strong chamomile tea can be applied to relieve the appearance of tired, puffy eyes.

Chamomile is used in natural hair, skin, & face care treatments.

Part Used:
Flowers

Side Effects:
Chamomile may not be recommended for use by women who are pregnant or nursing.

Chamomile is not recommended for use by women who have a hormone sensitive condition like endometriosis, fibroids, or certain types of cancer.

Chamomile is not recommended for use by people who are taking prescription blood thinners or suffering from a disorder where blood thinners are counter indicated.

Chamomile may cause an allergic reaction such as skin rashes, throat swelling, and shortness of breath in those who are allergic to plants in the ragweed family.

Additional uses and side effects may exist but further research is necessary to determine the exact properties and effects of use.

General:
Chamomile is native to Europe but has been naturalized as a landscape and herb plant in much of the word. Chamomile is easy to grow from seed. The flowering tops of the chamomile plant are used in tea, extract, and capsule form and can be applied whole to sooth skin conditions or chewed for mouth conditions. 2 tsp to 1 cup hot Distilled Water, steep 30 minutes. Up to 3 cups per day

The flowers of another species of chamomile Anthemis tinctoria known as dyer's chamomile yield a yellow toned colorant. Mordant – Alum

Chaparral
Chaparral, Creosote Bush, Greasewood, Hedionilla, Jarilla

Botanical Name:
Larrea tridentata

Common Uses:
Acne, Natural Skin Care – Burns, Eczema, Psoriasis

Traditional Use:
Chaparral tincture is used as a traditional ingredient in short term alcohol based topical treatments for acne, burns, contact dermatitis, eczema, and psoriasis

Part Used:
Flower, Leaf, Fruit

Side Effects:
Chaparral is not recommended for use by women who are pregnant or nursing.

Chaparral is for external use only – prolonged ingestion of chaparral can cause liver damage.

Chaparral is not recommended for long term use.

Chaparral may cause diarrhea, fever, headache, kidney damage, liver damage, nausea, stomach pain, weight loss, and allergic skin reactions.

Additional uses and side effects may exist but further research is necessary to determine the exact properties and effects of use.

General:
Chaparral is native to the Southwestern regions of the United States and Mexico where it is harvested for use as a tincture or traditional supplement up to 3 times daily.

Chickweed
Adder's Mouth, Chickweed, Star Chickweed, Starweed

Botanical Name:
Stellaria media

Common Uses:
Acne, Contact Dermatitis, Eczema, Psoriasis, Seborrhea

Traditional Use:
Chickweed is used as part of a cooling, anti-inflammatory ointment for conditions such as acne, eczema, hemorrhoids, and psoriasis.

Chickweed has been used in traditional topical ointment or poultice preparations to reduce the appearance of redness of the skin in conditions like seborrhea.

Part Used:
Flower, Leaf, Root, Stem

Side Effects:
Chickweed is cultivated as a kitchen herb and is generally considered safe for consumption.

Chickweed is not recommended for use beyond dietary by women who are pregnant or nursing.

Chickweed may cause diarrhea.

Chickweed may cause an allergic reaction or skin irritation in some people.

Additional uses and side effects may exist but further research is necessary to determine the exact properties and effects of use.

General:

Chickweed is native to Asia and Europe but has naturalized throughout much the world and is considered a weed by some. The leaves have been used as a cold vegetable and the whole plant has been used in traditional supplements treat a variety of ailments in tea and poultice applications.

Chlorophyll
Botanical Name:
Chlorophyll

Common Uses:
Natural Skin Care – Acne, Healing, Wound Care

Traditional Use:
Chlorophyll has been used in traditional topical preparations to speed wound healing.

Chlorophyll has traditionally been used to cleanse the body, oxygenate blood, and encourage new cell growth.

Chlorophyll has been used as a component in natural skin care products designed to promote healing and maintain healthy, blemish free skin.

Part Used:
Extract

Side Effects:
Chlorophyll is not recommended for use by women who are pregnant or nursing.

Overuse of chlorophyll may cause abdominal cramps, diarrhea, or gastrointestinal upset.

Chlorophyll is not recommended for use without the advice of a physician or qualified herbalist.

Additional uses and side effects may exist but further research is necessary to determine the exact properties and effects of use.

General:
Chlorophyll is the green pigment found in plants and algae. Chlorophyll is extracted from the plant and used as a dietary supplement, cosmetic, and traditional liquid supplement.

Chrysanthemum
Chrysanthemum, Mum

Botanical Name:
Chrysanthemum morifolium, Dendranthema grandiflorum

Common Uses:

Acne

Traditional Use:
Chrysanthemum has been used as part of a traditional topical ointment, mask, or wash to alleviate acne, boils, and persistent skin sores.

Part Used:
Flower

Side Effects:
Chrysanthemum is not recommended for use by women who are pregnant or nursing.

Chrysanthemum may cause an allergic reaction in some people.

Additional uses and side effects may exist but further research is necessary to determine the exact properties and effects of use.

General:
Chrysanthemum is a perennial aromatic cultivated as a flowering herb in all regions of the world. The essential oils are extracted or the flowers are dried, powdered, and used as a traditional supplement tea or capsule supplement up to 3 times daily.

Cleavers
Barweed, Bedstraw, Catchweed, Cleavers, Cleaverwort, Eriffe, Gallium, Goose Grass, Gosling Weed, Grip Grass, Hayriff, Hedge Burs, Mutton Chops, Scratchweed

Botanical Name:
Galium aparine, Galium odoratum

Common Uses:
Acne, Eczema, Psoriasis

Traditional Use:
Cleavers tea is traditionally used as part of an external wash or internal infusion treatment to detoxify the body and alleviate acne, eczema, and psoriasis.

Cleavers has been used in natural skin care products to help tighten the skin and reduce sagging & wrinkling.

Part Used:
Flower, Juice, Leaf

Side Effects:
Cleavers is not recommended for use by women who are pregnant or nursing.

Cleavers may affect blood sugar.

Cleavers is not recommended for use by people who are on blood thinning medication or who have a bleeding disorder.

Additional uses and side effects may exist but further research is necessary to determine the exact properties and effects of use.

General:
Cleavers is native to Africa, Asia, Europe, North America, and South America and has traditionally been harvested during the flowering season for use in a tea infusion made with 1 teaspoon of cleavers in 1 cup of hot Distilled Water. Allow to steep. Use up to 3 times daily.

Clove
Clove, Ding Xiang, Girofle, Kreteks, Lavanga

Botanical Name:
Syzygium aromaticum

Common Uses
Acne

Traditional Use:
Clove has been used in traditional topical preparations to alleviate the pain & inflammation associated with some types of acne.

Part Used:
Flower, Leaf, Stem - Oil

Side Effects:
Clove is not recommended for use beyond dietary by women who are pregnant or nursing.

Clove is not recommended for use beyond dietary by people who are taking blood thinning medication or who have a bleeding disorder.

Clove oil is highly irritating to the skin and should be handled with caution.

Clove may cause an allergic reaction in some people.

Additional uses and side effects may exist but further research is necessary to determine the exact properties and effects of use.

General:
Clove is native to Indonesia but has been cultivated in many areas of the world preferring high moisture and plentiful sun. The flowers are picked and dried before blooming or the oils are extracted from the flowers for use in traditional aromatherapy or topical preparations.

Coconut Oil
Coco Palm, Coconut Palm, Coconut Oil

Botanical Name:
Cocos nucifera

Common Uses:
Natural Skin Care

Traditional Use:
Coconut oil is a light oil that softens and heals skin making it suitable for all skin and hair types. It creates a natural foaming action when used in skin and hair care treatments.

Coconut oil helps to exfoliate the outer layer of dead skin cells and may reduce fine lines and wrinkles and smooth the skin.

Part Used:
Seed Meat, Oil

Side Effects:
Coconut is not recommended for use beyond dietary by women who are pregnant or nursing.

Coconut oil may raise cholesterol or weight.

Additional uses and side effects may exist but further research is necessary to determine the exact properties and effects of use.

General:
Coconut Oil is extracted from the nut of the coconut palm and is used in cooking, skin care, and traditional supplements.

Cowslip
Common Names:
Aretyke, Arthetica, Buckels, Butter Rose, Cowslip, Crewel, Drelip, Fairy Caps, Fairy Cup, Herb Perter, Key Flower, Mayflower, Paigle, Palsywort, Password, Peagle, Petty Mulleins, Plumrocks, Primrose, Primula

Botanical Name:
Primula veris

Common Uses:
Acne

Traditional Use:
Cowslip has been used in topical preparations to help clear the skin of blemishes and is traditionally given as a part of a cleaning scrub for acne.

Cowslip has been used as a traditional tea to help reduce the impurities in the body and as a treatment component for severe acne.

Part Used:
Flower, Leaf, Root

Side Effects:
Cowslip is not recommended for use by women who are pregnant or nursing.

Cowslip is not recommended for use by people who are on blood thinning medication or who have a bleeding disorder.

Cowslip may affect blood pressure and the ability to control blood pressure.

Cowslip may cause an allergic reaction in some people.

Overuse may cause gastrointestinal upset in some people.

General:
Cowslip is native to Asia and Europe where the roots and flowers are harvested, dried and incorporated into a traditional tea supplement given up to 3 times daily.

Crab Claw

Botanical Name:
Peperomia pellucida

Common Uses:
Acne

Traditional Use:
Crab Claw has been used as part of a traditional topical preparation to alleviate skin infections and some types of acne.

Part Used:
Leaf, Juice, Stem

Side Effects:
Crab Claw is not recommended for use by women who are pregnant or nursing.

Crab Claw may cause an allergic reaction or asthma like symptoms in some people.

Additional uses and side effects may exist but further research is necessary to determine the exact properties and effects of use.

General:
Crab Claw is native to Asia and South America but is cultivated in other regions where it has been used as a cooked supplement vegetable and harvested for traditional topical and supplement preparations.

Cypress
Botanical Name:
Cupressus sempervirens

Common Uses:
Acne, Natural Skin Care

Traditional Use:
Cypress oil is used in to reduce excess oils in skin and hair care products and has been added to treatments for certain types of acne.

Cypress is known to tighten skin and refine the appearance of pores making it useful in facial care products.

Part Used:
Needles, Twigs

Side Effects:
Cypress is not recommended for use by women who are pregnant or nursing.

Additional uses and side effects may exist but further research is necessary to determine the exact properties and effects of use.

General:
Cypress is a well known essential oil native to Turkey but cultivated in other regions where the needles and twigs are harvested for their oil.

Damask Rose
Botanical Name:
Rosa damanscena

Common Uses:
Acne, Eczema, Natural Skin Care, Seborrhea

Traditional Use:
Damask Rose is included in natural skin care preparations to help clear the complexion, hydrate the skin and alleviate skin irritation like acne, eczema, and seborrhea.

Part Used:
Bud, Oil

Side Effects:
Additional uses and side effects may exist but further research is necessary to determine the exact properties and effects of use.

General:

Damask Rose is a deciduous member of the Rose family cultivated for rich rose scent. The shoots and buds are harvested and eaten as a raw or cooked vegetable while the petals have been used as a cooked jam component. The buds are harvested for use as a traditional supplement or the oils are extracted for use as an aromatherapy component

Dandelion
Blowball, Cankerwort, Clock Flower, Cochet, Dandelion, Dudhal, Endive, Fairy Clock, Fortune Teller, Irish Daisy, Lion's Tooth, Priest's Crown, Puff Ball, Swine Snout, Wild Endive

Botanical Name:
Taraxacum officinale

Common Uses:
Acne, Eczema, Psoriasis

Traditional Use:
Dandelion root helps the body to dispose of excess bacteria, toxins and hormones and has traditionally been used to help relieve skin conditions like acne, eczema, and psoriasis.

Part Used:
Leaf, Flower, Root

Side Effects:
Dandelion is not recommended for use by women who are pregnant or nursing.

Dandelion is not recommended for use by people with gall bladder disease without the guidance of a physician or qualified herbalist.

Dandelion is not recommended for use by people with stomach ulcers or gastritis.

Dandelion may cause stomach upset and diarrhea in some people.

Dandelion may cause an allergic reaction in some people.

General:
Dandelion is native to Asia, Europe, and North America where it is considered an invasive weed growing easily in a variety of sun, soil, and moisture conditions. It has been used by a variety of societies as a supplement treatment including the Native Americans. Dandelion leaf, flower, and root are used in salads, teas, and extracts and the flowers are sometimes used to make wine or in traditional teas up to 3 times daily.

Dock – Bloody

Bloody Dock, Red Veined Dock

Botanical Name:
Rumex sanguineus

Common Uses:
Acne, Eczema, Psoriasis, Wound Care

Traditional Use:
Bloody Dock has been used as a traditional topical preparation to alleviate the symptoms of skin diseases like acne, eczema, and psoriasis.

Part Used:
Root

Side Effects:
Bloody Dock is not recommended for use by women who are pregnant or nursing.

Bloody Dock is not recommended for use by people with gout, rheumatism, arthritis, or kidney stones.

Additional uses and side effects may exist but further research is necessary to determine the exact properties and effects of use.

General:
Bloody Dock is a hardy perennial found growing in untended areas. The young leaves have been harvested for use as a cold or cooked vegetable and the leaves are harvested in the spring, dried and powdered for use in traditional supplements.

Dog Rose

Botanical Name:
Rosa canina

Common Uses:
Natural Skin Care

Traditional Use:
Dog Rose hip infusions are used as an astringent wash for sensitive skin.

Part Used:
Hip

Side Effects:
Additional uses and side effects may exist but further research is necessary to determine the exact properties and effects of use.

General:
Dog Rose is a deciduous shrub cultivated in many regions of the world. The hips are harvested, eaten raw or cooked, used in jams & syrups, or made into a nutritive tea. The hips are also dried & powdered

for use as a traditional topical or supplement preparation.

Dragon's Blood
Dragons Blood, Sangre

Botanical Name:
Daemonorops draco

Common Uses:
Acne, Eczema, Wound Care

Traditional Use:
Dragons' Blood has been used in traditional topical preparations to alleviate acne and eczema.

Dragon's Blood is a red colorant used as a dye product and ink component.

Dragon's Blood has traditionally been used as a topical balm or poultice component to prevent infection & speed healing of skin ulcers.

Dragon's Blood has been used as part of a traditional topical preparation to reduce the chance of infection, stop bleeding, and speed healing in wounds.

Part Used:
Bark, Resin

Side Effects:
Dragon's Blood is not recommended for use by women who are pregnant or nursing.

Additional uses and side effects may exist but further research is necessary to determine the exact properties and effects of use.

General:
Dragon's Blood is the resin of the Dragon Tree found in many tropical and sub-tropical regions around the world. The resin is harvested from the ripe fruit for use as a color varnish, dye product, and both commercial pharmaceuticals and traditional supplements where the active compound are extracted in an alcohol bath. Do not confuse Dragon's Blood Daemonorops draco with Dragon's Blood Croton lechleri.

Dulse
Crannach, Dillisk, Dilsk, Dulse, Red Algae, Sea Lettuce, Distilled Water Leaf

Botanical Name:
Rhodymenia palmata

Common Uses:

Acne, Eczema, Psoriasis

Traditional Use:
Dulse has been used as a traditional supplement to detoxify the body and alleviate certain skin conditions like acne, eczema, and psoriasis.

Part Used:
Leaf, Whole

Side Effects:
Dulse is not recommended for use by women who are pregnant or nursing.

Dulse is not recommended for use by people with hyperthyroidism.

Additional uses and side effects may exist but further research is necessary to determine the exact properties and effects of use.

General:
Dulse is a type of algae found on the coasts of both the Atlantic and Pacific oceans. It is harvested for use as a vegetable in some regions or for use in commercial supplements or traditional supplements.

Edelweiss
Edelweiss, Lion's Paw, Queen's Flower

Botanical Name:
Leontopodium alpinum

Common Uses:
Natural Skin Care, Wound Care

Traditional Use:
Edelweiss contains anti-oxidants and sun screening properties making it a common ingredient in natural skin care products.

Edelweiss has traditionally been used in topical ointments to promote cell regeneration and speed wound healing.

Side Effects:
Additional uses and side effects may exist but further research is necessary to determine the exact properties and effects of use.

General:
Edelweiss can be found growing in higher altitudes and is cultivated as an ornamental for disinfectant and supplement uses.

Elderberry

Baccae, Black Elder, Elder, Elderberry, Ellanwood, Ellhorn, European Alder, Holunderbeeren, Sambucus, Sauco, Sureau

Botanical Name:
Sambucus nigra

Common Uses:
Acne, Natural Skin Care

Traditional Use:
Elderberry has been used as part of a traditional supplement to help detoxify the body and alleviate skin conditions like acne.

Elderberry is used as part of natural skin care products to detoxify and tone the skin while helping to fight aging.

Part Used:
Berry

Side Effects:
Elderberry is not recommended for use by women who are pregnant or nursing.

Unripe or uncooked elder berries are toxic and may cause nausea, vomiting, and diarrhea.

Additional uses and side effects may exist but further research is necessary to determine the exact properties and effects of use.

General:
Elder is native to Europe and North America but has been cultivated in other regions. The dried flowers and cooked berries of the elder are traditionally used in teas, extracts, and capsule form with a traditional infusion preparation being 2 teaspoon of dried flower to 1-cup boiling Distilled Water 8 times daily.

Elder – Mexican
Botanical Name:
Sambucus mexicana

Common Uses:
Acne, Natural Hair & Skin Care

Traditional Use:
Mexican Elder flowers have been used as part of a traditional facial wash to alleviate acne outbreaks.

Part Used:
Flower, Root

Side Effects:
Mexican Elder is not recommended for use by women who are pregnant or nursing.

Mexican Elder may cause gastrointestinal upset.

Additional uses and side effects may exist but further research is necessary to determine the exact properties and effects of use.

General:
Mexican Elder is a deciduous shrub native to southern United States and Mexico where the flowers and fruit are harvested for use as a cooked or raw food product. The fruits and stems are used as dye products and the flower & root are harvested for use in traditional supplements.

Elecampane
Alant, Aster, Elecampane, Elfdock, Elfwort, Horse Elder, Horseheal, Indian Elecampane, Scabwort, Velvet Dock, Wild Sunflower, Yellow Starwort

Botanical Name:
Inula helenium

Common Uses:
Acne, Contact Dermatitis, Poison Ivy

Traditional Use:
Powdered Elecampane is traditionally added to a wash for the treatment of many eruptive skin diseases including acne, poison ivy, and boils.

Part Used:
Flower, Rhizome, Root

Side Effects:
Elecampane is not recommended for use by women who are pregnant or nursing.

Elecampane may cause allergies to people sensitive to plants in the sunflower family.

Elecampane may irritate the mucus membranes.

Elecampane may affect blood sugar.

Additional uses and side effects may exist but further research is necessary to determine the exact properties and effects of use.

General:
Elecampane is a perennial native to Europe and growing 4-6 feet in height that was naturalized to North America by the colonists and grows easily from root cuttings or seed. Elecampane prefers partial sunlight and moderate to highly moist soil. The root is harvested in the autumn, air dried, and ground or made in an alcohol extract for inclusion in traditional supplement preparations.

Elm - Indian
Indian Elm, Moose Elm, Orme Gras, Red Elm, Slippery Elm, Sweet Elm

Botanical Name:
Ulmus fulva

Common Uses:
Acne, Contact Dermatitis, Eczema, Wound Care

Traditional Use:
Indian Elm is traditionally included in topical ointments to draw impurities, reducing the appearance of acne and to treat eczema.

Indian Elm has a high mucilage content making it a traditional balm or poultice for burned, sun damaged, or irritated skin.

Indian Elm has been used as a traditional topical poultice to help speed healing in skin ulcers and wounds. It acts as a drawing ingredient to draw splinters, fragments, and infection away from the skin.

Part Used:
Flower, Inner Bark, Leaf

Side Effects:
Indian Elm is not recommended for use by women who are pregnant or nursing.

Indian Elm bark was once moistened and inserted into the vagina to cause cervical dilation and induce abortions.

Indian Elm may cause an allergic reaction.

Additional uses and side effects may exist but further research is necessary to determine the exact properties and effects of use.

General:
Indian Elm is native to North America and mature trees contain the highest level of active ingredients. The mature bark is harvested, dried, and ground fine for use in traditional supplement teas at a typical rate of rate of 2 tablespoons of powder to 1 cup of hot Distilled Water or base up to 3 times daily. Chopped root or liquid extracts are more commonly used in poultice preparations.

Fennel
Biri Sanuf, Bitter Fennel, Carosella, Fennel, Hinojo, Sweet Fennel, Wild Fennel, Xiao Hui Xiang

Botanical Name:
Foeniculum vulgare

Common Uses:
Acne, Natural Skin Care

Traditional Use:
Fennel has been used as a traditional supplement to increase urinary output and to help remove toxins from the body alleviating conditions like acne, gout, rheumatism and as a general detoxification agent.

Fennel oils have a natural cleansing and toning effect on the skin and are used in natural products to combat oil, fight wrinkles, and brighten the complexion.

Part Used:
Leaf, Oil, Root, Seed, Whole

Side Effects:
Fennel is not recommended for use by women who are pregnant or nursing.

Fennel is a uterine stimulant.

Fennel may cause photosensitivity, indigestion, pulmonary edema, and vomiting.

Fennel is not recommended for use by women who have an estrogen sensitive disorder like endometriosis, fibroids or certain types of cancer.

Additional uses and side effects may exist but further research is necessary to determine the exact properties and effects of use.

General:
Fennel is an annual plant native to the Mediterranean but is cultivated worldwide as it is easily grown from seed in rich soil with plenty of sun and moderate moisture. It grows to a height of 3-6 feet and has yellow flowers that bloom in the summer months. Fennel is harvested for use as a flavoring in beverages or dried and powdered for use in traditional supplements. The oils are extracted from the crushed seed for use in topical and aromatherapy treatments.

Figwort
Carpenter's Square, Figwort, Heal All, Scorphula

Botanical Name:
Scrophularia nodosa

Common Uses:
Acne, Detoxification, Eczema, Psoriasis, Wound Care

Traditional Use:

Figwort tea is traditionally used a detoxifier to reduce acne, eczema, and psoriasis outbreaks.

Figwort is a traditional ingredient in ointments and poultices that reduce pain & inflammation and help speed healing in eczema, psoriasis, and wounds.

Part Used:
Flower, Leaf, Root, Stem

Side Effects:
Figwort is not recommended for use by women who are pregnant or nursing.

Figwort is not recommended for use by people with heart disease.

Figwort may affect blood sugar.

Additional uses and side effects may exist but further research is necessary to determine the exact properties and effects of use.

General:
Figwort is native to North America, Europe, and China where it is harvested before flowering for use as a tincture traditionally delivered at a rate of 15 drops up to 3 times a day.

Fireweed
Blood Vine, Blooming Sally, Flowering Willow, French Willow, Purple Rocket, Rosebay, Tame Withy, Wickup, Willow Herb

Botanical Name:
Chamerion angustifolium

Common Uses:
Acne, Wound Care

Traditional Uses:
Fireweed has been used in traditional topical washes, ointments, and poultices to help reduce inflammation and reduce the appearance of acne.

Fireweed is used as a topical preparation to help draw infection from wounds or foreign matter from wounds.

Parts Used:
Flower, Leaf, Stem

Side Effects:
Fireweed is not recommended for use by women who are pregnant or nursing.

Additional uses and side effects may exist but further research is necessary to determine the exact properties and effects of use.

General:
Fireweed is native to North America where the above ground parts are harvested early in the season for use as a candied product, tea substitute, or cold vegetable.

Fumitory
Beggary, Earth Smoke, Fumaria, Fumitory, Fumus, Hedge Fumitory, Vapor, Wax Dolls

Botanical Name:
Fumaria officinalis

Common Uses:
Acne, Dermatitis, Eczema, Natural Skin Care – Pigmentation, Psoriasis

Traditional Use:
Fumitory is traditionally used as a skin wash for clearing conditions like acne, eczema, and psoriasis.

Fumitory is used as a traditional supplement to detoxify the body and helps to clear skin conditions like acne, eczema, and psoriasis.

Fumitory is used as part of a traditional preparation to reduce hyper-pigmentation like age spots, freckles and dark scarring.

Part Used:
Flower, Leaf, Stem

Side Effects:
Fumitory is not recommended for use by women who are pregnant or nursing.

Overuse of Fumitory may cause diarrhea, trembling, convulsions and even death.

Additional uses and side effects may exist but further research is necessary to determine the exact properties and effects of use.

General:
Fumitory is native to Africa, Europe, and Siberia but has been naturalized to parts of North & South America where it is harvested for use as a grated, fresh supplement.

Galbanum
Botanical Name:
Ferula galbaniflua

Common Uses:
Natural Skin Care, Wound Care

Traditional Uses:
Galbanum oil has been used to help regenerate aged skin and provide hydration in natural skin care products.

Parts Used:
Bark, Root - Resin

Side Effects:

Additional uses and side effects may exist but further research is necessary to determine the exact properties and effects of use.

General:
Galbanum resin is harvested from the roots and trunk of the tree for use as a food flavoring, cosmetic fragrance, and traditional supplement

Garlic Mustard
Alliaria petiolata

Common Uses:
Acne, Eczema, Wounds

Traditional Use:
Garlic Mustard has been used as a traditional detoxification to remove impurities and reduce the number and severity of acne and eczema attacks.

Garlic Mustard has been used as a traditional topical poultice or ointment to clean and speed healing in skin ulcers, wounds, and sores.

Part Used:
Leaf, Seed

Side Effects:
Additional uses and side effects may exist but further research is necessary to determine the exact properties and effects of use.

General:
Garlic Mustard is native to Africa and Asia but has been naturalized to Europe and North America where it is considered an invasive species by some. The young leaves are harvested as a seasoning or raw vegetable. The seeds are harvested for use in traditional supplements.

Geranium
Botanical Name:
Pelargonium graveolens

Common Uses:

Acne, Anti-Aging, Contact Dermatitis, Eczema, Natural Skin & Hair Care, Wound Care

Traditional Use:
Geranium has analgesic, anti-inflammatory, antimicrobial, astringent, and styptic properties that make it a traditional treatment for minor abrasions, cuts, & burns and for natural skin care remedies to treat acne, eczema, and contact dermatitis.

Germanium oil is used in natural skin care products for its effect on mature skin and the radiant glow it leaves on all skin types.

Part Used:
Leaf, Oil

Side Effects:
Geranium is not recommended for use, even in topical preparations, by women who are pregnant or nursing.

Geranium oil may cause an allergic reaction or skin irritation in some people.

Additional uses and side effects may exist but further research is necessary to determine the exact properties and effects of use.

General:
Geranium is native to South Africa but has been cultivated as an annual landscape herb in many other countries and is easily propagated by cuttings or seed. The oils are extracted from the leaves and stems through steam distillation and used in traditional inhalant therapy, supplements, and perfumes.

Golden Seal
Eye Balm, Eye Root, Goldenroot, Goldenseal, Ground Raspberry, Indian Dye, Indian Plant, Indian Turmeric, Jaundice Root, Orange Root, Turmeric Root, Wild Curcuma, Yellow Indian Pain, Yellow Puccoon, Yellow Root

Botanical Name:
Hydrastis canadensis

Common Uses:
Acne, Eczema, Psoriasis, Wound Care

Traditional Use:
Goldenseal is traditionally used in topical antiseptic and antibacterial ointments for minor abrasions, cuts, and open wounds. The ointment will also be anti-inflammatory and has been used as a traditional topical preparation in the treatment of skin conditions like acne and eczema.

Golden seal is traditionally used to cleanse the body of toxins including excess uric acid and toxins related to conditions like acne, gout & rheumatism.

Part Used:
Leaf, Root, Underground Stem

Side Effects:
Goldenseal is not recommended for use by women who are pregnant or nursing.

Goldenseal is not recommended for use in children's treatments.

Goldenseal is not intended for long-term use.

Goldenseal contains alkaloids that are toxic in large doses.

Overdose of goldenseal can cause vomiting, diarrhea, or stomach upset in some people.

Goldenseal may lower blood sugar levels, raise blood pressure, or gastrointestinal upset.

Goldenseal may change the way your body reacts to other prescription drugs.

Additional uses and side effects may exist but further research is necessary to determine the exact properties and effects of use.

General:
Goldenseal is native to North America and can be found growing wild in part of the US or cultivated in many supplement gardens. The leaf and the underground stem and root of the Goldenseal plant are harvested, dried, and powdered for use in supplement teas or made into an extract.

Goose Grass
Goose Grass, Moor Grass, Prince's Feather, Silverweed, Trailing Tansy, Wild Agrimony

Botanical Name:
Potentilla anserina

Common Uses:
Contact Dermatitis, Seborrhea, Skin Inflammation

Traditional Uses:
Goose Grass is traditionally applied to the skin to help reduce inflammation and irritation and helps to dry out sores in contact dermatitis like poison ivy.

Goose Grass tea has been used as a traditional skin cleansing lotion helping to alleviate inflammation, redness, and seborrhea.

Goose Grass has traditionally been bruised and applied directly to skin ulcers and hemorrhoids to alleviate pain & inflammation, reduce seepage & bleeding, and speed healing.

Parts Used:
Flower, Leaf

Side Effects:
Goose Grass is not recommended for use by women who are pregnant or nursing.

Additional uses and side effects may exist but further research is necessary to determine the exact properties and effects of use.

General:
Goose Grass grows worldwide and can be found growing in nearly every soil, sun & moisture conditions where some consider it an invasive weed. The root is harvested and eaten as a raw or cooked vegetable or dried & powdered for use as a thickening & flour product while the leaves are harvested early in the season for use fresh or dried in traditional supplements.

Gotu Kola
Brahma Buti, Centellase, Divya, Gotu Kola, Indian Pennywort, White Rot

Botanical Name:
Centella asiatica

Common Uses:
Acne, Contact Dermatitis, Eczema, Natural Hair & Skin Care, Psoriasis, Scar Reduction, Wound Care

Traditional Use:
Gotu Kola is an astringent and anti-inflammatory making it a traditional ingredient in skin care washes for the treatment of acne, eczema, psoriasis, and contact dermatitis.

Gotu Kola has traditionally been used as a balm to help sooth burns, skin ulcers, and wounds while speeding healing.

Gotu Kola is traditionally used to speed wound healing, stimulate collagen production, and helps reduce scarring from acne and wounds.

Gotu Kola tea is used in natural skin care products to strengthen and rejuvenate the skin, hair, and nails by stimulating collagen synthesis.

Part Used:
Leaf, Stem

Side Effects:
Gotu Kola is not recommended for use by women who are pregnant or nursing.

Gotu Kola is not recommended for use by people with liver disease.

High doses of Gotu Kola may cause nausea, rash, and possibly liver damage.

Do not use Gotu Kola if you are taking prescription drugs to treat depression, high cholesterol, or high blood pressure.

Additional uses and side effects may exist but further research is necessary to determine the exact properties and effects of use.

General:
Gotu Kola is native to Asia, Africa, North America and South America where it can be found growing in moist areas. The whole plant is harvested, dried in full sun, and used in traditional supplement teas and as a liquid extract up to 3 times daily.

Grapefruit
Agume, Grapefruit, Shaddock

Botanical Name:
Citrus paradisi

Common Uses:
Acne, Natural Hair & Skin Care, Preservative

Traditional Use:
Grapefruit seed oil is traditionally used in natural hair & skin care products to reduce oil, tone the skin and in treatments for some types of acne.

Grapefruit oil acts as a natural preservative in homemade cosmetics and supplements helping to extend their shelf life.

Part Used:
Fruit, Rind, Seed

Side Effects:
Grapefruit is not recommended for use beyond dietary in women who are pregnant or nursing.

Grapefruit may change the way that the body uses estrogen and is not recommended for use by menopausal women or by those who have an estrogen related condition like fibroids, endometriosis or certain types of cancer.

Grapefruit oil may cause photosensitivity.

Additional uses and side effects may exist but further research is necessary to determine the exact properties and effects of use.

Grape
Calzin, Draksha, Grape, Grape Seed, Grapeseed, Red Vine, Uva

Botanical Name:
Vitis vinifera

Branch, Leaf, Seed: Anti-Inflammatory, Anti-Viral, Astringent, Colorant, Diuretic, Emollient, Vasodilator

Common Uses:
Natural Hair & Skin Care

Traditional Use:
Grapeseed oil has emollient, regenerative and toning properties and is often used as a carrier oil in natural skin and hair care

Part Used:
Fruit, Leaf, Seed - Oil

Side Effects:
Grape is not recommended for use beyond dietary by women who are pregnant or nursing.

Grape seed may cause dizziness, dry scalp, high blood pressure, hives, indigestion, nausea, sore throat, stomach upset, and vomiting.

Additional uses and side effects may exist but further research is necessary to determine the exact properties and effects of use.

General:
The leaves, branches, and fruits of the grape have been used as a supplement since the time of the Ancient Greeks and the grapes used to produce grape seed extract are typically obtained from wine manufacturers.

The roots of another species of grape the wild grape, Vitis riparia roots yield a purple colorant.

Green Osier
Agoda Dogwood, Green Osier

Botanical Name:
Cornus alternifolia

Common Uses:
Acne, Contact Dermatitis, Eczema, Wound Care

Traditional Use:

Green Osier barks has traditionally been used as a powder or wash to reduce inflammation and help speed the healing of acne, blisters, eczema, and wounds.

Part Used:
Bark

Side Effects:
Additional uses and side effects may exist but further research is necessary to determine the exact properties and effects of use.

General:
Green Osier is native to North America where it has been used as a dye product and traditional supplement for thousands of years.

Guggul
Guggul, Koushika, Mukul Myrrh Tree

Botanical Name:
Commiphora wightii

Common Uses:
Acne

Traditional Uses:
Guggul has been used as a traditional supplement tea to help alleviate some types of acne and eczema outbreaks. Studies show that it may work as well as prescription antibiotics to reduce the number and severity of acne outbreaks.

Parts Used:
Resin

Side Effects:
Guggul is not recommended for use by women who are pregnant or nursing.

Guggul is not recommended for use by people who have a hormone sensitive condition like endometriosis, fibroids, or cancer.

Guggul is not recommended for use by people who have a thyroid condition.

Guggul may cause diarrhea, headaches, nausea, vomiting, or skin rashes in some people.

Additional uses and side effects may exist but further research is necessary to determine the exact properties and effects of use.

General:
Guggal is made from the gum resin of the Indian Mukul Tree. Guggal is cultivated for the gummy resin. It is harvested for use as a perfumery and incense similar to myrrh. The resin of Guggal has been used in traditional supplements since ancient times.

Gum Dragon
Adragante, Goat's Thorn, Green Dragon, Gum Dragon, Gummi Tragacanthae, Gum Tragacanth, Hog Gum, Tragacanto

Botanical Name:
Astragalus gummifera , Syrian Tragacanth

Common Uses:
Natural Care Products

Traditional Uses:
Dragon gum is used as a binding and thickening agent in toothpaste, hand lotion, creams, ointments, and jelly.

Parts Used:
Gum Resin

Side Effects:
Dragon Gum is not recommended for use beyond dietary by women who are pregnant or nursing.

Dragon Gum may cause an allergic reaction in some people.

Additional uses and side effects may exist but further research is necessary to determine the exact properties and effects of use.

General:
Gum Dragon is a plant whose resin is used as a cold-Distilled Water stabilizing and thickening agent in foods, pharmaceuticals, and personal care products. The resin is also used in supplement preparations.

Harts Tongue
Buttonhole, God's Hair, Hind's Tongue, Horse Tongue

Botanical Name:
Asplenium scolopendrium

Common Uses:
Acne, Natural Hair & Skin Care

Traditional Uses:
Harts tongue fronds have been used in natural hair & skin care washes to reduce oils and is traditionally believed to reduce acne.

Parts Used:
Leaf, Stem

Side Effects:
Harts tongue is not recommended for use by women who are pregnant or nursing.

Harts tongue is not recommended for long-term use.

Additional uses and side effects may exist but further research is necessary to determine the exact properties and effects of use.

General:
Harts tongue is an evergreen groundcover and harvested for use in natural hair & skin care products or traditional supplements.

Hawthorn
Aubepine, Haw, Hawthorne, Maybush, Maythorn, Whitehorn

Botanical Name:
Crataegus laevigata

Common Uses:
Acne, Eczema, Psoriasis

Traditional Uses:
Hawthorn berries have been used as a traditional treatment to reduce impurities and alleviate skin conditions like acne, eczema, and psoriasis.

Parts Used:
Berry, Flower, Leaf

Side Effects:
Hawthorn is not recommended for use by women who are pregnant or nursing.

Hawthorn is not recommended for use by people on medication for heart disease, blood pressure, or who have a condition related to heart or blood pressure. Hawthorn may change the way the body reacts to medications including digitalis.

Hawthorn can cause agitation, dizziness, fatigue, headache, insomnia, nausea, nosebleeds, and other problems in some people.

Additional uses and side effects may exist but further research is necessary to determine the exact properties and effects of use.

General:
Hawthorn is native to temperate northern regions where it has been used for hundreds of years as a food and traditional supplement. The berries, flowers, and leaves all contain active cardiac compounds but the most effect is found in the leaves harvested during the flowering season. Hawthorn is harvested, dried & powdered or available in commercial supplements.

Hazel
Aveleira, Cobnut, Hazel, Hazel Nut, Noisettes

Botanical Name:
Corylus avellana

Common Uses:
Carrier Oil, Natural Skin Care

Traditional Uses:
Hazelnut Oil is traditionally used in oily or combination natural hair & skin care products for its ability to tone and tighten the skin while promoting cell regeneration and infusing moisture.

Hazelnut has been used as a traditional dietetic additive to help lower cholesterol.

Hazelnut bark, roots, and nuts yield colorants in shades of brown to tan.

Hazelnut oil is traditionally used to treat intestinal parasites like threadworm.

Parts Used:
Bark, Leaf, Nut – Oil

Side Effects:
Hazelnut is not recommended for use beyond dietary by women who are pregnant or nursing.

Hazelnut may cause an allergic reaction in some people.

Additional uses and side effects may exist but further research is necessary to determine the exact properties and effects of use.

General:
Hazelnuts are the fruit of the hazel tree and are harvested as a food. Nuts are eaten whole, dried & powdered as a flour product, or included as a flavoring in drinks and foods. The nuts are also harvested for oil extraction and used as traditional supplements.

Hearts Ease
Field Pansy, Heartsease, Heart's Ease, Johnny Jump In, Ladies Delight, Pansy, Pennsee, Viola, Wild Pansy

Botanical Name:
Viola tricolor

Common Uses:

Acne, Eczema, Psoriasis

Traditional Use:
Hearts Ease is most traditionally used as an external ointment to help heal chronic skin conditions including acne, cradle cap, eczema, impetigo, and psoriasis.

Part Used:
Flower, Leaf, Stem

Side Effects:
Hearts Ease is not recommended for use by women who are pregnant or nursing.

Additional uses and side effects may exist but further research is necessary to determine the exact properties and effects of use.

General:
Hearts Ease is a member of the viola family native to Asia and Europe and cultivated in other regions where it is harvested during the flowering season, dried, and powdered for use in ointments, shampoos and traditional supplement teas up to 3 times daily.

Heartseed Walnut
Heartseed Walnut, Japanese Walnut

Botanical Name:
Juglans ailanthifolia cordiformis

Common Uses:
Acne, Natural Skin Care, Wound Care

Traditional Use:
The oils of the heartseed walnut are used in natural skin care products giving a light astringent and toning effect traditionally used to combat acne while smoothing the overall texture of the skin.

The oils of the heartseed walnut are used as a traditional topical preparation to speed healing in skin ulcers and minor wounds.

Part Used:
Nut - Oil

Side Effects:
Additional uses and side effects may exist but further research is necessary to determine the exact properties and effects of use.

General:
Heart Seed Walnut is a deciduous tree native to Asia where the seeds are harvested for use as a raw or cooked food product or the oils extracted for use in cooking or cosmetics.

Heather
Culluna, Heather, Ling

Botanical Name:
Calluna vulgaris

Common Uses:
Acne

Traditional Use:
Heather has traditionally been used to detoxify the body and lessen the severity and number of acne outbreaks.

Part Used:
Flower, Leaf

Side Effects:
Heather is not recommended for use by women who are pregnant or nursing.

Additional uses and side effects may exist but further research is necessary to determine the exact properties and effects of use.

General:
Heather is an evergreen shrub like plant growing 12-18 inches in height but able to be cultivated into a hedge. Heather blooms in mid-summer with a variety of pink toned flowers. It has been naturalized to the east coast of North America where it harvested while in bloom, dried and used as a traditional supplement tea up to 3 times daily.

Hemp Agrimony

Botanical Name:
Eupatorium cannabinum

Common Uses:
Acne

Traditional Use:
Hemp Agrimony has traditionally been used to detoxify the body and minimize the episodes of conditions like acne, gout, and rheumatism.

Part Used:
Flower, Leaf

Side Effects:
Hemp Agrimony is not recommended for use by women who are pregnant or nursing.

Hemp Agrimony contains compounds that make it unsuitable for use without the guidance of a physician or qualified herbalist.

Overuse of Hemp Agrimony may cause diarrhea, vomiting, or liver damage.

Additional uses and side effects may exist but further research is necessary to determine the exact properties and effects of use.

General:
Hemp Agrimony is native to Asia but cultivated as an ornamental plant in other regions where the flower & leaf are harvested, dried, and powdered for use in traditional supplements.

Henna
Alcanna, Egyptian Privet, Henna, Mehndi, Mendee, Mignonette Tree, Reseda, Smooth Lawsonia

Botanical Name:
Lawsonia inermis

Common Uses:
Acne, Eczema, Natural Hair & Skin Care,

Traditional Use:
Henna has illustrated an ability to ease the discomfort and appearance of skin conditions including acne, eczema, and psoriasis.

Part Used:
Bark, Fruit, Leaf

Side Effects:
Henna is not recommended for use by women who are pregnant or nursing.

Henna has been used as a uterine stimulant and may have abortifacient properties.

Henna is not recommended for use in children's treatments.

Henna is not recommended for internal treatments without the advice of a physician or qualified herbalist.

Henna may cause an allergic reaction or skin irritation.

Additional uses and side effects may exist but further research is necessary to determine the exact properties and effects of use.

General:
Henna is native to the Middle East where it is harvested, dried, and powdered for use in external applications or as a traditional supplement tea up to 3 times daily.

Honey Locust
Botanical Name:
Gleditsia sinensis

Common Uses:
Acne, Eczema, Psoriasis, Wound Care

Traditional Use:
Honey Locust thorns & thorns have traditionally been used as an ointment or wash to help clean & speed healing in acne, eczema, psoriasis and eruptive skin diseases.

Honey Locust juice & thorns have been used as a traditional skin wash or ointment to clean and speed healing of skin ulcers, sores, and wounds.

Part Used:
Leaf, Seed, Thorn

Side Effects:
Honey Locust may contain toxic compounds and is not recommended for use without the advice of a physician or qualified herbalist.

Honey Locust is not recommended for use by women who are pregnant or nursing.

Additional uses and side effects may exist but further research is necessary to determine the exact properties and effects of use.

General:
Honey Locust is a deciduous tree native to Asia, Europe and North America where the seedpod has been harvested for use as a soap product, the seeds have been used as a sugar substitute, and the wood is used for construction. The leaf, seed, and thorn are harvested for use in traditional supplements.

Honeysuckle – Japanese
Botanical Name:
Lonicera japonica

Common Uses:
Acne

Traditional Use:
Japanese Honeysuckle flowers & leaves have been used as a traditional topical preparation to alleviate certain types of acne outbreaks.

Part Used:
Bark, Flower, Leaf

Side Effects:

Japanese Honeysuckle is not recommended for use by women who are pregnant or nursing.

Additional uses and side effects may exist but further research is necessary to determine the exact properties and effects of use.

General:
Japanese Honeysuckle is native to Asia and is commonly cultivated in many regions of the world as a fragrant and ornamental. Japanese Honeysuckle has been used in Chinese supplements for thousands of years. The leaves are harvested and eaten as a cooked vegetable while the flowers are used as a sweet syrup.

Horse Chestnut - Indian
Botanical Name:
Aesculus indica

Common Uses:
Acne, Eczema, Psoriasis

Traditional Use:
Indian Horse Chestnut oil has traditionally been used as a topical wash or ointment ingredient to alleviate acne, eczema, and psoriasis.

Part Used:
Seed - Oil

Side Effects:
Indian Horse Chestnut is not recommended for use by women who are pregnant or nursing.

Indian Horse Chestnuts are known to have narcotic properties and should not be used without the advice of a physician or qualified herbalist.

Additional uses and side effects may exist but further research is necessary to determine the exact properties and effects of use.

Houseleek
Ayegreen, Bullock's Eye, Hens and Chicks, Jupiter's Beard, Thunder Plant

Botanical Name:
Sempervivum tectorum

Common Uses:
Acne, Eczema, Psoriasis

Traditional Uses:
Houseleek has been used as a traditional topical or supplement preparation to alleviate itchy or eruptive skin conditions like acne, eczema, and psoriasis.

Houseleek is traditionally included as part of a topical ointment to cleanse and speed healing in burns, sores, skin ulcers, and wounds.

Houseleek juice has been used as a traditional topical preparation to remove warts & corns.

Parts Used:
Whole - Juice

Side Effects:
Houseleek is not recommended in women who are pregnant or nursing.

General:
Houseleeks are a form of evergreen succulent found in higher altitudes worldwide where they are cultivated in sunny rock gardens and for use as a traditional supplement. The plant is harvested and juiced for use in topical preparations and the leaves are used as part of a traditional supplement.

Hyacinth
Bai Qu, Hyacinth - Orchid

Botanical Name:
Bletia hyacinthina

Common Uses:
Acne, Eczema, Psoriasis, Skin Damage, Wounds

Traditional Use:
Hyacinth bulb is traditionally powdered for use in topical preparations to attract moisture, reduce itching & inflammation, and speed healing in conditions like acne, burns, eczema, psoriasis, skin damage, and wounds.

Part Used:
Bulb - Root

Side Effects:
Hyacinth is not recommended for use by women who are pregnant or nursing.

Additional uses and side effects may exist but further research is necessary to determine the exact properties and effects of use.

General:
Hyacinth is native to Japan but is also a common ornamental cultivated worldwide for its spring flowers. The bulb is used to add sheen to ink, polishes, and other products and as a traditional supplement.

Immortelle

Shrubby Everlasting, Eternal Flower, Goldilocks, Immortelle, Sandy Everlasting, Strawflower, Yellow Chaste Weed

Botanical Name:
Helichrysum angustifolium

Common Uses:
Anti-Aging, Natural Skin Care, Scar Reduction

Traditional Use:
Immortelle is believed to have regenerative properties that stimulate new skin cell production making it a common ingredient in skin care treatments especially for aged skin.

Immortelle is a traditional component in natural skin care treatments to reduce the appearance of cellulite and fade the appearance of hyperactive pigmentation, scarring, and stretch marks.

Part Used:
Flower

Side Effects:
Immortelle is not recommended for use by women who are pregnant or nursing.

Immortelle is not recommended for use in children's treatments.

Immortelle is not recommended for use by people who have a blocked bile duct or gallstones.

Immortelle may cause an allergic reaction in some people.

Additional uses and side effects may exist but further research is necessary to determine the exact properties and effects of use.

General:
Immortelle is native to Europe and the United States and is harvested as the buds begin to bloom. They are dried, powdered and used in traditional supplement teas up to 3 times daily. Immortelle oil is steam distilled within 24 hours of harvesting the flower for use in topical and aromatherapy preparations.

Indian Coral
Flame Tree, Indian Coral, Kaffirboom

Botanical Name:
Erythrina variegata

Common Uses:
Acne, Eczema, Psoriasis, Wound Care

Traditional Use:
Indian Coral is used as a traditional topical preparation to reduce inflammation and speed healing of acne, eczema, psoriasis, wounds, and other inflammatory skin conditions.

Part Used:
Bark, Leaf

Side Effects:
Indian Coral is not recommended for use by women who are pregnant or nursing.

Additional uses and side effects may exist but further research is necessary to determine the exact properties and effects of use.

General:
Indian Coral is a flowering tree cultivated in tropical and subtropical regions for its showy flowers. The leaves and bark have been harvested for use in traditional topical and supplement preparations.

Indian Mallow
Abutilon, Dong Kui Zi, Indian Mallow

Botanical Name:
Abutilon indicum

Common Uses:
Acne, Wound Care

Traditional Use:
Indian Mallow has been used as a traditional topical poultice to reduce the pain & inflammation while speeding healing in acne, skin ulcers, and wounds.

Part Used:
Whole Plant – Bark, Flower, Leaf, Root, Stem

Side Effects:
This is not recommended for use by women who are pregnant or nursing.

Additional uses and side effects may exist but further research is necessary to determine the exact properties and effects of use.

General:
Indian Mallow is a shrub native to tropical and sub-tropical regions where it is cultivated as an ornamental and the whole plant is harvested, dried, and powdered for use as a traditional supplement infusion.

Indigo – Wild

American Indigo, Baptista, False Indigo, Horsefly Weed, Indigo Broom, Rattlebush, Wild Indigo, Yellow Indigo

Botanical Name:
Baptisia tinctoria

Common Uses:
Acne, Wound Care

Traditional Use:
Wild Indigo has traditionally been used as part of a topical ointment, wash, or poultice to treat infections like staphylococcus, reduce acne outbreaks, and speed healing in skin ulcers and wounds.

Part Used:
Root

Side Effects:
Wild Indigo is not recommended for use by women who are pregnant or nursing.

Wild Indigo is not recommended for use in children's treatments.

Wild Indigo is not recommended for people with gastrointestinal disorders.

Overuse of Wild Indigo may cause diarrhea, difficulty breathing, increased heart rate, nausea, vomiting or even death.

Additional uses and side effects may exist but further research is necessary to determine the exact properties and effects of use.

General:
Wild Indigo is native to North America where it can be found growing wild along the Eastern half of the country. It is harvested, dried and powdered for use in traditional supplement infusions up to 3 times daily or in ointment preparations at a rate of 1:1 in 60% alcohol.

Iris – Yellow
Iris, Yellow Flag, Yellow Iris

Botanical Name:
Iris pseudacorus

Common Uses:
Acne, Wound Care

Traditional Use:
Yellow Flag is traditionally used to reduce inflammation, pain, and speed healing in severe acne, skin ulcers, and wounds.

Part Used:
Root

Side Effects:
Yellow Iris is not recommended for use by women who are pregnant or nursing.

Yellow Iris may cause an allergic reaction or skin irritation.

Overuse of Yellow Iris may cause severe diarrhea and vomiting.

Additional uses and side effects may exist but further research is necessary to determine the exact properties and effects of use.

General:
Yellow Iris is a scented perennial cultivated as an ornamental in many regions of the world. The seed is harvested for use as a coffee substitute and the flowers & roots are used as a dye product. The root is used to make ink and in traditional supplements.

Irish Moss

Botanical Name:
Chondrus crispus

Common Uses:
Acne, Natural Hair & Skin Care Products, Skin Inflammation

Traditional Use:
Irish Moss has traditionally been used as a topical ointment or wash component to alleviate acne and skin inflammation.

Part Used:
Whole

Side Effects:
Irish Moss is not recommended for use by women who are pregnant or nursing.

Additional uses and side effects may exist but further research is necessary to determine the exact properties and effects of use.

General:
Irish Moss is a red algae that is collected from the coast of Ireland, washed, bleached in the sun, and powdered for use as a thickening agent, stabilizer, and as a traditional supplement infusion.

Ivy - English

English Ivy, Gum Ivy, Lierre Grimpant, True Ivy, Woodbind

Botanical Name:
Hedera helix

Common Uses:
Acne, Wound Care

Traditional Use:
English Ivy has been used in topical ointments and washes to help reduce the appearance of acne outbreaks.

Part Used:
Berry, Leaf

Side Effects:
English Ivy is not recommended for use by women who are pregnant or nursing.

English Ivy may cause an allergic reaction or gastrointestinal upset in some people.

Additional uses and side effects may exist but further research is necessary to determine the exact properties and effects of use.

General:
English ivy is native to Asia and Europe but has been naturalized to many areas of the world where it is harvested, dried, and powdered for use in external applications or traditional tea supplement up to 3 times daily.

Jasmine
Jasmine, Jessamine

Botanical Name:
Jasminum officinale

Common Uses:
Natural Skin & Hair Care

Traditional Use:
Jasmine Oil is included in natural hair & skin care products to help tone dry or greasy skin and promote elasticity.

Part Used:
Flower, Oil – pick before dawn when oils are strongest
Side Effects:
Jasmine is not recommended for use by women who are pregnant or nursing.

Additional uses and side effects may exist but further research is necessary to determine the exact properties and effects of use.

General:
Jasmine is cultivated in many regions of the world as an ornamental plant but is also harvested for use as a traditional tea or oil supplement. Jasmine flower are traditionally harvested at dawn when the oils are strongest.

Jojoba
Deernut, Goatnut, Jojoba, Pignut

Botanical Name:
Simmondsia chinensis

Common Uses:
Acne, Carrier Oil, Natural Hair, Skin & Face Care, Preservative, Psoriasis

Traditional Use:
Jojoba helps to unclog the pores and dissolve excess sebum and is traditionally used in topical preparations to alleviate some types of acne.

Jojoba is a rich, moisturizing oil that resembles the sebum in human skin and is easily absorbed by the skin and does not cause irritation for most skin types making it a preferred oil for use in natural hair & skin care products.

Jojoba has been used as a natural preservative in supplements, food products, and cosmetics.

Part Used:
Leaf, Seed, Oil, Wax

Side Effects:
Jojoba Oil is for external use only and should not be ingested.

Jojoba may cause an allergic skin reaction in some people.

Additional uses and side effects may exist but further research is necessary to determine the exact properties and effects of use.

General:
Jojoba is native to the Deserts of North America and Latin America. The oil and wax produced by the Jojoba seed are used in natural care products and supplements.

Jurema
Botanical Name:
Mimosa hostilis

Common Uses:
Acne, Burns, Natural Skin Care, Wounds

Traditional Use:
Jurema is used in commercial and traditional skin care products to rejuvenate the skin, reduce acne, and combat aging.

Jurema is traditionally used in topical preparations to reduce pain, speed healing, and rejuvenate skin in injuries like burns, sores, ulcers, and wounds.

Part Used:
Leaf

Side Effects:
is not recommended for use by women who are pregnant or nursing.

Additional uses and side effects may exist but further research is necessary to determine the exact properties and effects of use.

General:
Jurema is an evergreen shrub native to Central America and South America where it has been harvested as a traditional supplement for thousands of years.

Juniper
Guinevere, Ginepro, Juniper, Juniper Berries, Zimbro

Botanical Name:
Juniperus communis

Common Uses:
Acne, Eczema, Psoriasis, Wound Care

Traditional Use:
Juniper oil has astringent and antiseptic properties that make it a traditional toning oil for acne treatments while its stimulating properties have shown benefits in treating eczema and psoriasis.

Part Used:
Berry, Needles, Oil

Side Effects:
Juniper is not recommended for use by women who are pregnant or nursing.

Juniper is not recommended for use by people who have diabetes, intestinal disorders, high blood pressure or kidney disease.

Overuse may cause urine to smell like violets.

Overdose can cause kidney irritation, blood in the urine, and potential liver damage.

Juniper Oil is for external use only.

Additional uses and side effects may exist but further research is necessary to determine the exact properties and effects of use.

General:
Juniper is native to Africa, Asia, Europe and North America. Juniper berries are harvested for use as a diet or tea supplement while the oils are extracted from the needles. Do not bruise or crush the berries until you are ready to use them.

Kokum
Botanical Name:
Garcinia indica

Common Uses:
Contact Dermatitis, Eczema, Skin Irritation

Traditional Use:
Kokum leaves & bark have been used as a traditional infusion or topical preparation to alleviate skin irritation, eczema, and contact dermatitis.

Part Used:
Bark, Fruit, Leaf

Side Effects:
Kokum is not recommended for use by women who are pregnant or nursing.

Additional uses and side effects may exist but further research is necessary to determine the exact properties and effects of use.

General:
Kokum is a fruit bearing tree native to Africa, Asia, and India where it is cultivated for a variety of uses. The fruit is harvested as a food or drink product, the oils are harvested for use in foods, medicines, and cosmetics, and the bark, leaf, and fruit are used as commercial pharmaceuticals, traditional supplements and dietary supplements.

Kombu
Kombu, Konbu

Botanical Name:
Laminaria japonica

Common Uses:
Natural Hair & Skin Care

Traditional Use:
Kombu has been used as a natural hair & skin care product to provide essential nutrition, remove toxins

and give a silky smooth feel to the hair, lips, nails, and skin.

Part Used:
Whole

Side Effects:
Kombu is not recommended for use by women who are pregnant or nursing.

Kombu is not recommended for use by people with a thyroid disorder and may cause thyroid changes in others.

Kombu is not recommended for use by people who have a kidney disorder.

Additional uses and side effects may exist but further research is necessary to determine the exact properties and effects of use.

General:
Kombu is a seaweed cultivated in Asia for use as a nutritious food or harvested, dried, and powdered for use in traditional supplements.

Kukui Nut
Candlenut, Indian Walnut, Kukui Nut, Varnish Tree

Botanical Name:
Aleurites moluccanus

Common Uses:
Acne, Eczema, Mouth Natural Hair & Skin Care, Psoriasis, Wound Care

Traditional Use:
Kukui nut oil is able to penetrate deep into the skin and scalp and is often used in treatments for dry, damaged skin & hair, to fade scars, to alleviate acne, eczema and psoriasis.

Kukui nut oil is high in Vitamins A, C, E, linoleic acids, and fatty acids and provides anti-oxidants that help to heal and protect the skin making it a traditional topical preparation for treating skin sores, ulcers, and wounds.

Side Effects:
Kukui nut is not recommended for use by women who are pregnant or nursing.

Kukui nut may cause an allergic reaction in some people.

Additional uses and side effects may exist but further research is necessary to determine the exact properties and effects of use.

General:
Kukui nut has been naturalized over nearly every tropical and sub-tropical region of the world. The nut is used as a food, the oils are used as a wood and fiber product varnish and the inner bark yields a dye product used as ink and for cosmetic purposes. The nuts have been used as a body & hair soap.

Kwao Kreu
Botanical Name:
Pueraria mirifica

Common Uses:
Hyper-Pigmentation

Traditional Use:
Kwao Kreu is traditionally used as a topical preparation to reduce hyper-pigmentation like age spots, scarring, and freckles.

Side Effects:
Kwao Kreu is not recommended for use by women who are pregnant or nursing.

Kwao Kreu is not recommended for use by women who have a hormone sensitive condition like endometriosis, fibroids, and certain types of cancers.

Additional uses and side effects may exist but further research is necessary to determine the exact properties and effects of use.

General:
Kwao Kreu is native to Thailand and cultivated in other regions where it has been used as a traditional supplement and commercial supplement.

Labrador Tea
Botanical Name:
Ledum groenlandicum

Common Uses:
Acne, Eczema, Contact Dermatitis, Wound Care

Traditional Use:
Labrador tea leaves have traditionally been used in topical washes & ointments to speed healing and reduce irritation in skin conditions like acne, eczema, and contact dermatitis.

Labrador tea leaves have been included in traditional topical preparations to speed healing in skin sores, ulcers, and wounds.

Part Used:

Leaf

Side Effects:
Labrador Tea is not recommended for use by women who are pregnant or nursing.

Labrador Tea may develop narcotic toxins if allowed to ferment in a closed container for an extended period.

Additional uses and side effects may exist but further research is necessary to determine the exact properties and effects of use.

General:
Labrador tea is made from the leaves of an evergreen shrub found growing naturally in northern climates. The leaves have been used as a refreshing tea, flavoring, and insect repellant.

Lady's Fingers
Kidney Vetch, Lady's Fingers, Woundwort

Botanical Name:
Anthyllis vulneraria

Common Uses:
Acne, Eczema, Wound Care

Traditional Use:
Lady's Fingers have traditionally been used as a wash or ointment in speeding healing and skin regeneration in acne, eczema, skin sores, ulcers, and slow healing wounds.

Part Used:
Leaf, Root

Side Effects:
This is not recommended for use by women who are pregnant or nursing.

Additional uses and side effects may exist but further research is necessary to determine the exact properties and effects of use.

General:
Lady's Fingers are native to Asia and Europe but has been naturalized to North America where it can be found growing wild in grasslands and mountainous regions. The flowers, leaves, and roots are harvested during flowering, dried, and powdered for use in traditional topical preparations.

Lavender
Botanical Name:
Lavandula angustifolia, Lavendula officinalis

Common Uses:
Acne, Natural Hair & Skin Care

Traditional Use:
Lavender is a core ingredient in many oily skin and acne treatments to help reduce blemishes and kill bacteria. Lavender blends well with astringent carrier oils like grapeseed.

Part Used:
Flower, Leaf, Stem

Side Effects:
Lavender is not recommended for use by women who are pregnant or nursing.

There have been reports that topical use of lavender oil can cause breast growth in boys, men, and young women.

Lavender may cause changes in appetite, constipation, headaches and drowsiness in some people.

Lavender can cause skin irritation in some people.

Lavender is not recommended for use with anti-anxiety, anti-depressants, antihistamines, or sedatives.

Overuse of lavender oil for internal supplements can be toxic if taken by mouth. Oils are for external use only. The leaves can be ingested.

Additional uses and side effects may exist but further research is necessary to determine the exact properties and effects of use.

General:
Lavender is native to the Mediterranean and was used in supplements and ceremonial treatments in ancient Egypt, Greece, and Rome. Lavender is cultivated worldwide for use as a traditional aromatherapy, supplement tea, or extract.

Lemon
Botanical Name:
Citrus limonum

Common Uses:
Acne, Natural Hair & Skin Care

Traditional Use:
Lemon oil helps to brighten dull complexions and is a gentle cleanser for oily skin and hair. The cleansing and antibacterial properties make it a traditional choice for acne treatments. Lemon is also an astringent and is often included in masks to

help refresh the skin and prevent the formation of wrinkles.

Lemon oil is traditionally used as a poultice or traditional supplement to strengthen capillaries and help reduce the appearance of varicose veins.

Part Used:
Juice, Rind - Oil

Side Effects:
Lemon is not recommended for use beyond dietary by women who are pregnant or nursing.

Lemon oil is phototoxic oil and should not be used in skin or hair treatments when the user will be exposed to sunlight.

Lemon oil should be diluted when using in any remedy as it may irritate the skin.

Additional uses and side effects may exist but further research is necessary to determine the exact properties and effects of use.

General:
Lemon is native to India but has been cultivated around the world where it is harvested for use in culinary, supplement, cosmetic, and cleaning recipes.

Lemongrass
Citronella, Fever Grass, Lemon Grass, Lemongrass

Botanical Name:
Cymopogon citratus

Common Uses:
Acne, Enlarged Pores, Natural Skin & Hair Care

Traditional Use:
Lemongrass has antibacterial, anti-inflammatory, and astringent properties that make it a traditional ingredient in treating acne and reducing the appearance of large pores.

Lemongrass helps to detoxify the system removing impurities in treatments for acne.

Lemongrass reduces excess oils in skin and hair and is often included in natural shampoos, facial washes, ointments and toners.

Part Used:
Leaf, Stalk, Oil

Side Effects:

Lemon grass is not recommended for use by women who are pregnant or nursing.

Lemon grass may cause an allergic reaction or skin irritation.

Additional uses and side effects may exist but further research is necessary to determine the exact properties and effects of use.

General:
Lemon Grass is native to Asia but is now cultivated in many regions of the world where the stalks are harvested for use as a highly nutritious food and the leaves & oils are harvested and prepared as a traditional supplement tea or essential oil.

Lime
Botanical Name:
Citrus aurantifolia

Common Uses:
Acne, Natural Skin Care

Traditional Use:
Lime is added to creams to help clear the skin of toxins & oils helping to reduce acne.

Lime is sometimes used as a replacement for lemon in natural hair & skin care recipes.

Part Used:
Oil, Peel

Side Effects:
Lime is not recommended for use beyond dietetic by women who are pregnant or nursing.

Lime oil may cause photosensitivity in some people.

Additional uses and side effects may exist but further research is necessary to determine the exact properties and effects of use.

General:
Lime is native to Asia but is cultivated in other semi-tropic regions where it is harvested for consumption and use in supplements.

Logwood
Bloodwood, Logwood

Botanical Name:
Haematoxylon campechianum

Common Uses:
Skin Pigmentation

Traditional Use:
Logwood is believed to reduce the amount of pigmentation in the skin and is often used in preparations to prevent or reduce freckles, dark scars, and age spots.

Part Used:
Heart Wood

Side Effects:
Logwood is not recommended for use by women who are pregnant or nursing.

Logwood is for external use only. Internal use of Logwood may cause fever, vomiting, and even death in some individuals.

Additional uses and side effects may exist but further research is necessary to determine the exact properties and effects of use.

General:
Logwood is native to North America, Mexico and Central America and is known as the spiny tree. It is used to give grey lavender to blue purple tones in dying or dried and powdered for use in external supplement preparations.

Macadamia Nut
Australian Nut, Bopple Nut, Bush Nut, Macadamia Nut, Queensland Nut

Botanical Name:
Macadamia tetraphylla

Common Uses:
Carrier Oil

Traditional Uses:
Macadamia Nut oil is an exceptionally light oil and is valued as a carrier oil especially for treatments for those with oily or sensitive skin.

Parts Used:
Nut

Side Effects:
Macadamia Nuts are not recommended for use beyond dietary by women who are pregnant or nursing.

Additional uses and side effects may exist but further research is necessary to determine the exact properties and effects of use.

General:
Macadamia Nuts are native to Australia but are cultivated commercially in other regions where they are harvested for use as a food.

Magnolia
Beaver Tree, Ho No Ki, Holly Bay, Hou Po, Indian Bark, Japanese Whitebark, Magnolia, Red Bay, Red Magnolia, Swamp Laurel, Swamp Sassafras, Sweet Bay, White bay, White Laurel, Xin Ye, Hua

Botanical Name:
Magnolia officinalis

Flower - Analgesic, Anti-Inflammatory, Colorant, Nervine, Sedative

Oil – Antiseptic, Stimulant

Common Uses:
Contact Dermatitis, Hyper-Pigmentation, Wound Care

Traditional Uses:
Magnolia bark and petal oils are traditionally used in topical washes or ointments to reduce itchiness in contact dermatitis and speed healing in skin sores, ulcers, & wounds.

Magnolia has been incorporated into treatments designed to reduce dark skin pigmentation including age spots, freckles, and scarring.

Parts Used:
Bark, Flower Bud

Side Effects:
Magnolia is not recommended for use by women who are pregnant or nursing.

Magnolia may cause heartburn, headaches, sleepiness or tremors.

Additional uses and side effects may exist but further research is necessary to determine the exact properties and effects of use.

General:
Magnolia is a scented ornamental cultivated in many warmer areas of the world. The petals & buds are harvested for use as a food or harvested at the beginning of the flowering season, dried, in the sun, and powdered for use in traditional supplements. The oil is also extracted from the petals by steam distillation for use in aromatherapy and traditional supplements. The bark is harvested for use in an alcohol extraction.

Mallow – Common
Common Mallow, High Mallow, Tall Mallow, Malva

Botanical Name:

Malva sylvestris

Common Uses:
Acne, Eczema, Psoriasis, Wound Care

Traditional Use:
Common Mallow has traditionally been used as a topical preparation to sooth inflammation and reduces the appearance of acne.

Common Mallow has traditionally been used as a poultice or ointment to sooth skin inflammation, speed healing and reduce seepage in eczema, psoriasis, sores, ulcers, and wounds.

Part Used:
Leaf

Side Effects:
Common Mallow is not recommended for use by women who are pregnant or nursing.

Common Mallow is not recommended for use by people who have an auto-immune disorder like lupus or multiple sclerosis.

Additional uses and side effects may exist but further research is necessary to determine the exact properties and effects of use.

General:
Common Mallow is native to Africa and Asia but has naturalized to Europe and North America. Common Mallow leaves are eaten as a cooked vegetable. Common Mallow is used as a gentler version of Marsh Mallow and is most commonly used fresh as a decoction.

Mallow – Little
Cheeseweed, Little Mallow

Common Uses:
Contact Dermatitis, Eczema, Natural Hair & Skin Care, Psoriasis, Wound Care

Traditional Use:
Little Mallow has been used in natural cosmetic products to soften and smooth the texture of skin and hair and to treat dandruff.

Little Mallow has traditionally been used as a poultice or ointment to sooth skin inflammation, ease pain, speed healing and reduce seepage in contact dermatitis, eczema, psoriasis, sores, ulcers, and wounds.

Part Used:
Leaf, Root, Seed

Side Effects:
Little Mallow is not recommended for use by women who are pregnant or nursing.

Additional uses and side effects may exist but further research is necessary to determine the exact properties and effects of use.

General:
Little Mallow is native to Africa and Asia but is now common to fields & untended areas in most regions of the world. The leaves are harvested for use as a raw or cooked vegetable and the leaves & roots are harvested for use fresh or dried in traditional supplements.

Mallow - Marsh
Althea, Mallards, Marsh Mallow, Marshmallow, Smart Weed, Wymote

Botanical Name:
Althaea officinalis

Common Uses:
Acne, Detoxification, Eczema, Psoriasis

Traditional Use:
Marshmallow root has been used as a traditionally topical preparation to help sooth inflamed skin and speed healing in conditions like acne, eczema, psoriasis, sores, and ulcers.

Marshmallow root has been used as a traditional supplement to bind toxins and detoxify the body in general health treatments and as a supplementary component for conditions like acne, eczema, and psoriasis.

Part Used:
Flower, Root

Side Effects:
Marsh Mallow is not recommended for use by women who are pregnant or nursing.

Marsh Mallow contains high levels of mucilage and pectin that might interfere with the absorption rate of some medications.

Marsh Mallow may lower blood sugar.

Additional uses and side effects may exist but further research is necessary to determine the exact properties and effects of use.

General:
Marsh Mallow is native to Europe but has been naturalized to many regions of the world including North America. Marsh Mallow root is most often

used as a food additive. The flowers are harvested during blooming and the root is harvested in the fall for use in traditional supplement teas or tinctures.

Mangosteen
Mangosteen, Queen of Fruits

Botanical Name:
Garcinia mangostana

Common Uses:
Acne

Traditional Uses:
Mangosteen has been used as a traditional supplement to treat certain types of acne by helping to stop the growth of acne causing bacteria.

Parts Used:
Fruit, Heartwood, Leaf, Juice, Rind

Side Effects:
Mangosteen is not recommended for use by women who are pregnant or nursing.

Additional uses and side effects may exist but further research is necessary to determine the exact properties and effects of use.

General:
Mangosteen is a fruit native to the tropical areas of the world where it is harvested as a food but is also used in commercial health drinks & supplements and traditional supplement preparations.

Manketti
Manketti, Mongongo

Botanical Name:
Schinziophyton rautanenii

Common Uses:
Natural Skin Care, Pigmentation – Scarring, Wound Care

Traditional Use:
Manketti oil is hydrating and regenerative and is used in natural skin care products especially for aged skin.

Manketti has traditionally been used in topical treatments to help speed healing in skin sores, ulcers, and wounds while preventing scarring.

Side Effects:
Manketti is not recommended for use by women who are pregnant or nursing.

Additional uses and side effects may exist but further research is necessary to determine the exact properties and effects of use.

General:
Manketti is native to Africa where the nuts are eaten as a food and the oil is harvested by steam distillation for use in cosmetics, aromatherapy, and traditional supplement treatments.

Mares Tail
Common Mare's Tail, Marestail

Botanical Name:
Hippuris vulgaris

Common Uses:
Acne, Wound Care

Traditional Use:
Marestail has been used as a traditional topical preparation to stop bleeding and speed healing in acne, skin sores, skin ulcers, and wounds.

Part Used:
Leaf

Side Effects:
Marestail is not recommended for use by women who are pregnant or nursing.

Additional uses and side effects may exist but further research is necessary to determine the exact properties and effects of use.

General:
Marestail is native to Europe and North America where it can be found growing in bogs & ponds where it is considered an invasive weed by some. The leaves are harvested for use as a fresh or cooked vegetable or used fresh or dried as a traditional supplement.

May Chang
May Chang, Tropical Verbena

Botanical Name:
Litsea cubeba

Common Uses:
Acne

Traditional Use:
May Chang has been used as a traditional topical preparation to reduce bacteria and alleviate the severity of acne outbreaks.

Part Used:
Fruit, Oil

Side Effects:
May Chang is not recommended for use by women who are pregnant or nursing.

May Chang is not recommended for internal use by people who have glaucoma or a similar disorder.

May Chang may cause an allergic reaction or skin irritation.

Additional uses and side effects may exist but further research is necessary to determine the exact properties and effects of use.

General:
May Chang is native to Asia and naturalized in other areas where the fruit for use or the oils are extracted by steam distillation for use as a traditional supplement or aromatherapy treatment.

Moneywort
Creeping Jenny, Creeping Joan, Herb Two Pence, Meadow Runagates, Moneywort, Running Jenny, Serpentaria, String of Sovereigns, Twopenny Grass, Wandering Jenny, Wandering Tailor

Botanical Name:
Lysimachia nummularia

Common Uses:
Acne, Eczema, Psoriasis, Wound Care

Traditional Use:
Moneywort has traditionally been used as a wash to ease acne outbreaks.

Moneywort's most common traditional use is as an external wash or ointment component to treat eczema and psoriasis and to help speed wound healing.

Part Used:
Whole

Side Effects:
Moneywort is not recommended for use by women who are pregnant or nursing.

Additional uses and side effects may exist but further research is necessary to determine the exact properties and effects of use.

General:
Moneywort is native to Europe and has been naturalized to North America and Japan where it is harvested while in bloom, dried, and powdered for use in a traditional supplement tea which is taken internally up to 3 times daily or incorporated into a topical preparation.

Myrrh
Botanical Name:
Commiphora myrrha

Common Uses:
Natural Skin Care, Wound Care

Traditional Use:
Myrrh resin is traditionally used as a topical preparation to speed healing in skin ulcers, cold sores, & canker sores.

Myrrh is believed to have rejuvenating and regenerative effects on the skin making it a common component in natural skin care products especially those designed to reduce scarring.

Part Used:
Resin

Side Effects:
Myrrh is not recommended for use by women who are pregnant or nursing.

Overuse of Myrrh can cause nausea or vomiting.

Myrrh may affect the menstrual cycles in some women.

Individuals with diabetes should consult with a physician before using myrrh as it may affect blood sugar.

Additional uses and side effects may exist but further research is necessary to determine the exact properties and effects of use.

General:
Myrrh is native to the Mediterranean but is cultivated in other regions where the resin is harvested during the summer months for use in perfumery and traditional supplements. The bark is wounded to cause a formation of oily resin that is harvested and the oils extracted by steam distillation.

Neem
Arishtha, Beard Tree, Holy Tree, Indian Lilac, Margosa, Neem

Botanical Name:
Azadirachta Indica

Common Uses:
Acne, Eczema, Natural Hair & Skin Care, Psoriasis, Wound Care

Traditional Use:
Neem leaf tea has been used as a traditional topical preparation to reduce bacterial, inflammation, and dryness associated with acne.

Neem has been used as a traditional topical preparation or soap & shampoo ingredient to relieve the itchiness, redness, and duration of acute eczema and psoriasis outbreaks.

Neem oil has moisturizing and regenerative properties among other components that make it a common ingredient in natural hair, skin, nail, & mouth care cosmetics alleviating conditions like dandruff, dry skin, itchy scalp and hyper pigmentation.

Neem has been used as a traditional topical preparation to reduce infection while speeding healing of skin sores, ulcers, and wounds.

Part Used:
Bark, Leaf, Seed Nut Oil

Side Effects:
Neem is not recommended for use by women who are pregnant or nursing.

Neem is not recommended for use in children's treatments not for internal use.

Neem is not recommended for use by people with an auto-immune disease like Multiple Sclerosis and Lupus.

Neem may lower blood sugar.

Large doses of Neem Oil can be toxic if taken internally – for external use only.

Overuse of Neem may cause diarrhea, drowsiness, loss of consciousness, coma and even death.

Additional uses and side effects may exist but further research is necessary to determine the exact properties and effects of use.

General:
Neem is native to the tropical regions of Africa and Asia where all parts of the tree are harvested. The shoots & flowers of the tree are harvested as a vegetable, the gum is used as a thickening agent, and the stems are used as a tooth cleaning brush. The seeds are harvested and the oil steam extracted or the barks & leaves are harvested, dried, & powdered for use in traditional supplements & cleaning products.

Oats
Avena, Green Oat, Oat, Oatgrass, Oatmeal, Oatstraw, Wild Oat

Botanical Name:
Avena sativa

Common Uses:
Eczema, Psoriasis

Traditional Use:
Oats are traditionally included in poultices and scrubs to sooth the inflammation associated with skin conditions like acne, contact dermatitis, eczema, psoriasis, and sunburns.

Part Used:
Leaf, Stem - Green

Side Effects:
Oats are not recommended for use beyond dietary by women who are pregnant or nursing.

Oats may cause a reaction in individuals who are sensitive to gluten.

Oats may lower blood sugar.

Oats may cause skin irritation in some people.

Additional uses and side effects may exist but further research is necessary to determine the exact properties and effects of use.

General:
Oats are cultivated in much of North America but are also found growing wild in gardens, fields, and elsewhere. Oats are harvested during the flowering season and used fresh in a traditional supplement tea or applied directly or as a tincture to the skin. Processed oats generally have little to no nutritional or supplement value. You should use fresh, green oats whenever attempting to attain the benefits of oat based treatments.

Olive
Acide Gras, Jaitun, Manzanilla Olive, Olive, Olive Leaf, Olive Oil

Botanical Name:
Olea europea

Common Uses:
Carrier Oil

Traditional Use:

Olive leaf extract has shown to have antioxidant and antimicrobial properties and may be a beneficial component in washes and ointments for disinfecting minor abrasions, cuts, and skin wounds.

Olive oil has long been used as part of natural hair & skin care recipes and is especially effective at treating skin irritation and providing essential nourishment for the hair and skin.

Part Used:
Leaf, Seed Oil

Side Effects:
Olive Oil is not recommended for use beyond dietary by women who are pregnant or nursing.

Olive Oil may cause an allergic reaction in some people.

General:
Olive is cultivated in many regions of the world where the leaves are harvested, shade dried, and used in traditional supplement infusions up to 4 times a day or as oil based dietary or supplement treatment.

Orange - Sweet
Botanical Name:
Citrus sinensis

Common Uses:
Acne, Natural Skin Care

Traditional Use:
Sweet Orange rind has been used as an exfoliating product to alleviate acne.

Part Used:
Oil, Rind

Side Effects:
Sweet Orange is not recommended for use beyond dietary by women who are pregnant or nursing.

Sweet Orange oils may cause increased pigmentation or photosensitivity.

Sweet Orange may cause an allergic reaction or skin irritation.

Additional uses and side effects may exist but further research is necessary to determine the exact properties and effects of use.

General:
Sweet Orange is commonly cultivated as a juice or fruit product, the rind is used as a flavoring and the

flowers are cooked as a vegetable or used as a tea product. The rind and oils have been used in cosmetics.

Orange
Botanical Name:
Citrus aurantium

Common Uses:
Natural Skin Care

Traditional Use:
Orange oil is often added to facial and skin care treatments to create a radiant glow and promote fresher, younger looking skin.

Part Used:
Fruit, Rind

Side Effects:
Orange is not recommended for use beyond dietary by women who are pregnant or nursing.

Additional uses and side effects may exist but further research is necessary to determine the exact properties and effects of use.

General:
Orange is commonly cultivated as a juice or fruit product, the rind is used as a flavoring and the flowers are cooked as a vegetable or used as a tea product. The rind and oils have been used in cosmetics, cleaners, and aromatherapy treatments.

Orris Root
Bearded Iris, Daggers, Flag, Flaggon, Flag Lily, Fliggers, Florentine Iris, Gladyne, Iris, Jacob's Sword, Liver Lily, Myrtle Flower, Orris Root, Poison Flag, Purple Flag, Queen Elizabeth Root, Shegg, Snake Lily, Distilled Water Flag, White Dragon Flower, Wild Iris, Yellow Flag, Yellow Iris

Botanical Name:
Iris germanica

Common Uses:
Natural Skin Care

Traditional Use:
Orris Root has a pleasant floral scent and is often used as a scent fixative in natural hair & skin care, household cleaning or perfumery products, and perfumes.

Part Used:
Rhizome Root

Side Effects:
Orris is for external use only. Ingestion may cause bloody stools, mouth irritation, stomach pain, and vomiting.

Orris is not recommended for use by women who are pregnant or nursing.

General:
Orris root is naturalized to the United States and can be found growing in a variety of soil, sun, and Distilled Water conditions. The root is harvested, dried, and powdered for use in traditional supplements, perfumes, cleaning, and cosmetic products.

Palmarosa
Indian Geranium, Palmarosa

Botanical Name:
Cymbopogon martinii

Common Uses:
Acne, Natural Skin Care, Wound Care

Traditional Use:
Palmarosa oil has antibacterial and astringent properties and is traditionally used to reduce excess oils & bacteria in skin conditions like acne.

Palmarosa oil is used in natural skin care products for its hydrating, regenerative, and balancing effect that leaves the skin supple while aiding in fighting wrinkles.

Palmarosa oil is used in traditional topical preparations to reduce infection and speed healing of skin sores, ulcers, and wounds.

Part Used:
Grass Oils

Side Effects:
Palmarosa oil is not recommended for use by women who are pregnant or nursing.

Palmarosa oil is for external use only.

Additional uses and side effects may exist but further research is necessary to determine the exact properties and effects of use.

General:
Palmarosa is a species of grass related to citronella grass native to Asia and India but cultivated in other regions for its essential oil. The oil is extracted through steam distillation for use in cosmetics, perfumes, and supplements.

Papaya
Melon Tree, Papaya

Botanical Name:
Carica papaya

Common Uses:
Natural Skin Care – Pigmentation, Scar Reduction

Traditional Use:
The milk of the papaya contains high levels of papain and is traditionally used in natural skin care products to remove age spots, freckles, and scarring.

Papaya fruit is traditionally included in poultice treatments to help reduce scar tissue and has been found to be especially effective in burn care.

Part Used:
Fruit, Leaf

Side Effects:
Papaya is not recommended for use beyond dietary by women who are pregnant or nursing.

Papaya can have a laxative effect.

Papaya leaf, fruit, and seeds contain an anti-parasitic alkaloid that could be dangerous in high doses.

Papaya may cause an allergic reaction or skin irritation.

Additional uses and side effects may exist but further research is necessary to determine the exact properties and effects of use.

General:
Papaya is native to Central and South America where the leaves are harvested early in the growing season and the fruit is harvested when it is ripe.

Patchouli
Huo Xiang, Patchouli, Patchouly, Puthca Pat

Botanical Name:
Pogostermon patchouli

Common Uses:
Acne, Eczema, Natural Skin Care, Skin Scarring, Wound Care

Traditional Use:
Patchouli is used in traditional topical preparations to help treat acne & eczema.

Patchouli is often used in natural skin care recipes for relief from dry, itchy skin and to promote healing.

Patchouli is used as a traditional topical preparation to stimulate cell regeneration, speed healing, and reduce scarring of skin sores, ulcers, and wounds.

Part Used:
Leaf Oil

Side Effects:
Patchouli is not recommended for use by women who are pregnant or nursing.

General:
Patchouli is native to India but can be cultivated worldwide as long as it is protected from frost. The easiest method of propagation is through cuttings. Patchouli Oil is extracted from the leaves for use in topical preparations.

Pea
Common Pea, Garden Pea, Green Pea, Pea

Botanical Name:
Pisum sativum

Common Uses:
Acne

Traditional Use:
Powdered peas have been used as a traditional mask or poultice ingredient to alleviate bacterial skin conditions like acne.

Part Used:
Seed

Side Effects:
Peas are not recommended for use beyond dietary by women who are pregnant or nursing.

Additional uses and side effects may exist but further research is necessary to determine the exact properties and effects of use.

General:
Peas are cultivated in gardens and commercial enterprises as a food product but are also dried & powdered for use as flour or traditional topical preparation or the oils extracted for use as a traditional supplement preparation.

Peach

Botanical Name:

Prunus persica

Common Uses:
Carrier Oil

Traditional Use:
Peach is used in natural hair & skin care products for its light moisturizing affect suitable for all skin types.

Part Used:
Bark, Leaf, Flower, Fruit, Kernel – Oil

Side Effects:
Peach is not recommended for use beyond dietary by women who are pregnant or nursing.

Additional uses and side effects may exist but further research is necessary to determine the exact properties and effects of use.

General:
Peach trees are native to Asia but have been naturalized in many other regions where the fruit is cultivated as a food.

Petitgrain
Botanical Name:
Petitgrain bigarade

Common Uses:
Acne, Natural Hair & Skin Care

Traditional Use:
Pettigrain is antibacterial and astringent making it a traditional ingredient in acne treatment washes.

Petitgrain oil is used in natural cosmetic products to combat oily skin and hair.

Part Used:
Leaf

Side Effects:
Petitgrain is not recommended for use by women who are pregnant or nursing.

Additional uses and side effects may exist but further research is necessary to determine the exact properties and effects of use.

General:
Petitgrain oil is extracted from the leaves or unripe fruit of the orange tree by steam distillation and is used in perfumery, aromatherapy, and traditional supplements.

Picao Preto

Broomstick, Picao Preto, Spanish Needle

Botanical Name:
Bidens pilosa

Common Uses:
Acne, Wounds

Traditional Use:
Picoa has traditionally been used as a topical preparation to treat bacterial infections like staphylococcus and to combat certain types of acne.

Picoa has been used as a traditional topical wash or ointment to reduce infection, stop bleeding, and speed healing in skin sores, ulcers, and wounds.

Part Used:
Whole

Side Effects:
Picoa is not recommended for use by women who are pregnant or nursing.

Additional uses and side effects may exist but further research is necessary to determine the exact properties and effects of use.

General:
Picao is native to many tropical regions and cultivated in many warmer areas where the shoots & leaves are eaten as a raw or cooked vegetable, or the whole plant is harvested for use as a traditional supplement infusion.

Pipsissewa
Ground Holly, Pipsissewa

Botanical Name:
Chimaphila umbellate

Common Uses:
Acne, Eczema

Traditional Use:
Pipissewa has been used as a traditional supplement to remove toxins from the body and reduce skin conditions like acne & eczema.

Part Used:
Leaf

Side Effects:
Pipsissewa is not recommended for use by women who are pregnant or nursing.

Additional uses and side effects may exist but further research is necessary to determine the exact properties and effects of use.

General:
Pipsissewa is a flowering evergreen native to much of the Northern Hemisphere where the leaves are harvested during the flowering season for use as a flavoring or dried and powdered for use as a traditional supplement.

Pomegranate
Dadima, Pomegranate

Botanical Name:
Punica granatum

Common Uses:
Eczema, Natural Hair & Skin Care, Psoriasis

Traditional Use:
Pomegranate oils are valued for their ability to treat dry skin, eczema, and psoriasis as well as their ability to moisturize and regenerate aging skin while reducing the appearance of fine lines & wrinkles. Some research is being conducted to determine if the tannins and other compounds found in pomegranate oils are of benefit in preventing the formation of UV induced skin cancer.

Part Used:
Bark, Fruit, Oil, Rind, Seed

Side Effects:
Pomegranate is not recommended for use by women who are pregnant or nursing.

Pomegranate bark extracts are very toxic. Do not use bark extracts.

Pomegranate may cause an allergic reaction in some people.

Additional uses and side effects may exist but further research is necessary to determine the exact properties and effects of use.

General:
Pomegranate is native to Africa, China, and India and has been naturalized to parts of California and Arizona easily propagated by seed it is cultivated as an ornamental plant in full sun and well-drained soil.

Psyllium
Botanical Name:
Plantago psyllium

Common Uses:
Natural Hair & Skin Care

Traditional Use:
Plantago psyllium seeds are a good source of fiber and can absorb up to 14 times its weight in Distilled Water making it a useful thickening agent in natural skin and hair care products.

Part Used:
Seed, Seed Husks

Side Effects:
Psyllium is not recommended for use by women who are pregnant or nursing.

Psyllium seeds should not be used with any other stimulant laxative.

Psyllium seeds may interfere with the absorption of essential minerals, nutrients, vitamins, and medications and is not for long term use.

Drink plenty of fluids whenever Psyllium is being used as a dietary or supplement component.

Additional uses and side effects may exist but further research is necessary to determine the exact properties and effects of use.

General:
Psyllium Seeds come from the Plantain plant native to many countries of the world and can be found growing wild in much of North America. The seeds are harvested for use as a cosmetic, dietary, or medicinal product.

Pumpkin Seed
Calabaza, Curcurbita, Pumpkin, Pumpkin Seed

Botanical Name:
Cucurbita pepo

Common Uses:
Natural Hair & Skin Care

Traditional Use:
Pumpkin seed oil is beneficial in healing dry, damaged skin including skin suffering from minor abrasions, cuts, and wounds.

Part Used:
Oil, Seed

Side Effects:
Pumpkin seeds & oil are not recommended for use women who are pregnant or nursing.

Pumpkin seed & oil may affect a developing fetus.

Pumpkin and Pumpkin Seed may cause indigestion and diarrhea in some individuals.

Additional uses and side effects may exist but further research is necessary to determine the exact properties and effects of use.

General:
Pumpkin seed is often dried and powdered and seed oil should be cold pressed and consumed uncooked as heat can minimize the beneficial properties.

Rabbitbrush
Botanical Name:
Ericameria nauseosa

Common Uses:
Acne, Wound Care

Traditional Use:
Rabbitbrush has been used in traditional topical preparations to reduce skin inflammations like acne and to speed healing of skin sores, ulcers, and wounds.

Part Used:
Stems, Twigs

Side Effects:
Rabbitbrush is not recommended for use by women who are pregnant or nursing.

Rabbitbrush is not recommended for internal use without the advice of a physician or qualified herbalist.

Overuse of Rabbitbrush may cause an extreme drop in blood pressure.

Additional uses and side effects may exist but further research is necessary to determine the exact properties and effects of use.

General:
Rabbitbrush is a shrub native to North America where it is cultivated as an ornamental or as a forage plant. The leaves have been used as a sanitary padding, the flower head as a stuffing material, and the root sap as a source of hypoallergenic rubber or gum product.

Radish
Botanical Name:
Raphanus sativus

Common Uses:
Acne, Natural Skin Care

Traditional Use:
Radish is traditionally used in topical preparations to remove excess oils related to oily skin and reduce the severity of certain types of acne outbreaks.

Part Used:
Leaf, Root, Seed

Side Effects:
Radish is not recommended for use beyond dietary by women who are pregnant or nursing.

Additional uses and side effects may exist but further research is necessary to determine the exact properties and effects of use.

General:
Radish is cultivated as a food source worldwide and is also harvested for traditional supplement use with 1 radish grated to a juice pulp and mixed in a base, steeped for 12-24 hours and used at a rate of 1 spoonful every hour until symptoms abate.

Ragweed
Giant Ragweed, Horseweed, Ragweed
Botanical Name:
Ambrosia trifida

Common Uses:
Acne, Contact Dermatitis

Traditional Use:
Ragweed leaf juices have been used in traditional topical preparations to treat bacterial infections and to reduce the severity of acne outbreaks.

Crushed Ragweed have been used as a topical preparation to alleviate the inflammation, itchiness, and seepage associated with conditions like insect bites, stings, and contact dermatitis like poison ivy.

Part Used:
Flower, Leaf

Side Effects:
Ragweed is not recommended for use by women who are pregnant or nursing.

Ragweed can cause severe allergic reactions in some people.

Additional uses and side effects may exist but further research is necessary to determine the exact properties and effects of use.

General:
Ragweed is considered a weed found growing throughout untended areas of North America but it was cultivated by the Native Americans as an oil producing plant and food product.

Raspberry
Framboise, Raspberry, Raspberry Leaf
Botanical Name:
Rubus idaeus

Common Uses:
Acne, Natural Hair & Skin Care, Wound Care

Traditional Use:
Raspberry leaves have shown an astringent and local anti-inflammatory effect making it a traditional ingredient for poultices, masks, and washes for the treatment of acne, hemorrhoids, and skin wounds.

Raspberry leaf has been used in traditional topical preparations to speed healing in skin sores, ulcers, and wounds.

Part Used:
Bark, Fruit, Leaf

Side Effects:
Raspberry Leaf Tea is not recommended for use by women who are pregnant or nursing.

Raspberry Leaf Tea is not recommended for use by women who have a hormone sensitive condition like endometriosis, fibroids or certain types of cancer.

Raspberry leaf may cause uterine contractions.

Use fully dried leafs as the leaf develops toxins during the drying process that can cause nausea in some people.

Additional uses and side effects may exist but further research is necessary to determine the exact properties and effects of use.

General:
Raspberry can be found in many regions of the world and is native to much of North America and Canada. Though raspberry can thrive in a variety of conditions, it does prefer partly shaded areas for optimal growth. The fruit is harvested as a food and the leaves are harvested, dried, powdered and incorporated into traditional supplement teas.

Ravensara
Botanical Name:

Ravensara Aromatica

Common Uses:
Acne, Wound Care

Traditional Use:
Ravensara has been used as a traditional topical preparation to reduce the severity of acne outbreaks and to treat bacterial infections.

Ravensara is used in traditional preparations to reduce the likelihood of infections in skin wounds.

Part Used:
Bark – Leaf – Oil

Side Effects:
Ravensara is not recommended for use by women who are pregnant or nursing.

Additional uses and side effects may exist but further research is necessary to determine the exact properties and effects of use.

General:
Ravensara is native to Madagascar and cultivated elsewhere for the essential oils extracted from the bark & leaves. The oils are extracted through steam distillation and used in topical and aromatherapy preparations.

Red Clover
Beebread, Cloveone, Cow Clover, Daidzeln, Meadow Clover, Purple Clover, Red Clover, Wild Clover
Botanical Name:
Trifolium pratense

Common Uses:
Acne, Eczema, Psoriasis

Traditional Use:
Red clover has traditionally been used as an external wash for relief from skin conditions like acne, eczema, and psoriasis.

Red Clover tea is given up to 3 times daily as a traditional supplement to help purify the blood in treatment plans for acne, arthritis, and gout.

Part Used:
Flower

Side Effects:
Red clover is not recommended for use by women who are pregnant or nursing.

Red clover is not recommended for use by women who have a hormone sensitive condition like endometriosis, fibroids, or certain types of cancer.

Red clover is not recommended for use by people with a bleeding disorder.

Red clover may have contraceptive effects by rendering the cervix less accessible to sperm entry and should not be used by anyone attempting to conceive.

Red clover may cause an allergic reaction or skin irritation.

Additional uses and side effects may exist but further research is necessary to determine the exact properties and effects of use.

General:
The flowers of the Red Clover are found in many regions of the world including Asia, Africa, Europe, North America, and South America. The leaves and flowering tops have been used in traditional supplement teas, tinctures, extracts, and powders. Red clover belongs to the legume family and is native to North America and can be found growing wild in open meadows and fields.

Rooibos
Green Bush Tea, Kaffree Tea, Red Tea, Red Bush Tea, Rooibos

Botanical Name:
Aspalathus linearis

Common Uses:
Acne, Eczema, Psoriasis

Traditional Use:
The anti-histamine ability of Rooibos has made it a traditional ingredient in teas to minimize reactive conditions like acne, asthma, eczema, psoriasis, and seasonal allergies.

Part Used:
Branch, Leaf

Side Effects:
Rooibos is not recommended for use by women who are pregnant or nursing.

Additional uses and side effects may exist but further research is necessary to determine the exact properties and effects of use.

General:
Rooibos is native to Africa where it is harvested, chopped, and allowed to sun dry for use as a tea.

Rooibos should be slow dried using only natural lighting. The tea is used as a traditional supplement.

Rose

Botanical Name:
Rosa centifolia

Common Uses:
Acne, Natural Skin Care – Inflammation, Wound Care

Traditional Use:
Rose petals and bark are used to make an astringent skin care wash that is traditionally used to reduce acne outbreaks, disinfect minor wounds, and speed the healing process of damaged skin.

Rose Distilled Water is often used as a facial toning ingredient and has anti-inflammatory compounds that may make it beneficial in treating skin inflammations including mild acne.

Part Used:
Bark, Flower - Oil

Side Effects:
Rose is not recommended for use by women who are pregnant or nursing.

Additional uses and side effects may exist but further research is necessary to determine the exact properties and effects of use.

General:
Roses are cultivated as an aromatic ornamental in most regions of the world. The highest supplement qualities can be found in non-hybrid roses whose tea and oils are a deep red tone.

Rosebay

Rhododendron, Rosebay, Snow Rose

Botanical Name:
Rhododendron aureum

Common Uses:
Acne, Bacterial Infections, Wound Care

Traditional Use:
Rosebay oil has traditionally been used as a topical ointment to alleviate certain types of acne.

Part Used:
Flower, Leaf, Stem

Side Effects:

Rosebay is not recommended for use by women who are pregnant or nursing.

Internal use of Rosebay may cause inebriation and is considered toxic.

Additional uses and side effects may exist but further research is necessary to determine the exact properties and effects of use.

General:
Rosebay is a shrub native to Asia & Europe and cultivated in mountainous regions where the flowers are harvested during flowering & dried for use as a traditional supplement while the flowers, leaves, and stems are harvested and the oils extracted through steam distillation for use in topical preparations

Rose – Eglantine

Rose – Eglantine, Sweet Briar

Botanical Name:
Rosa rubiginosa

Common Uses:
Natural Skin Care – Anti-Aging, Scar Reduction, Wound Care

Traditional Use:
Eglantine Rose petals are traditionally used to speed healing of skin sores, skin ulcers, and minor wounds.

Eglantine Rose seed oils are rich in vitamin E and have been used in natural skin care products to reduce the signs of aging, the appearance of scars and to speed healing of minor skin wounds.

Part Used:
Flower, Fruit, Seed – Oil

Side Effects:
Eglantine Rose is not recommended for use by women who are pregnant or nursing.

Eglantine Rose may cause mouth, throat, or gastro-intestinal irritation.

Additional uses and side effects may exist but further research is necessary to determine the exact properties and effects of use.

General:
Eglantine Rose is traditionally cultivated as an ornamental or hedge shrub. The fruit is harvested for use as a cooked jelly or vitamin rich tea product. The petals and shoots are eaten as a raw or cooked vegetable. The seeds have been

ground into powder and used as a flour nutritional supplement. Oils are steam extracted from the fruits & seeds for use in topical and supplement products.

Rose Geranium
Botanical Name:
Pelargonium odorantissimum

Common Uses:
Acne, Natural Skin Care

Traditional Uses:
Rose Geranium is a has a light citrus-rose scent that makes it a common ingredient in perfumed cosmetics and is traditionally used to help clear the skin of excess oil while promoting healing making it a common ingredient in skin care recipes for oily and acne prone skin.

Parts Used:
Leaf, Stem

Side Effects:
Rose Geranium is not recommended for use by women who are pregnant or nursing.

Rose Geranium may cause skin irritation.

Additional uses and side effects may exist but further research is necessary to determine the exact properties and effects of use.

General:
Rose Geranium is native to Africa and Egypt but is cultivated in many regions where the leaves are harvested at the end of the season and the oils extracted for use in perfumes and traditional medicinals.

Rose Hip
Common Uses:
Anti-Aging, Natural Skin Care

Traditional Uses:
Rose hip oils are naturally high in GLA, contain collagen stimulating compounds, and help to reduce fine lines and wrinkles while preventing scarring making them a common ingredient in natural skin & wound care products.

Parts Used:
Hip, Seed

Side Effects:
Rose Hips are not recommended for use by women who are pregnant or nursing.

Rosehips may affect blood sugar.

Overuse of rose hips may cause diarrhea, fatigue, heartburn, nausea, sleep interruption, and vomiting.

Rosehip oil may aggravate acne in some people.

Additional uses and side effects may exist but further research is necessary to determine the exact properties and effects of use.

General:
The rose hips are the rounded portion of the flower just below the petals and contain the seeds of the rose. The rose hip is dried, powdered and used in traditional supplement infusions or the oil is extracted by steam distillation for use in topical, aromatherapy, or traditional supplements.

Rosewood
Bois de Rosa, Rosewood

Botanical Name:
Aniba rosaeodora

Common Uses:
Natural Skin Care

Traditional Use:
Rosewood oil regenerates damaged skin while infusing moisture and is a beneficial component in many skin care treatments including creams, lotions, massage treatments, and soaps with an added benefit of a beautiful scent.

Part Used:
Bark – Oils

Side Effects:
Rosewood is not recommended for use by women who are pregnant or nursing.

Additional uses and side effects may exist but further research is necessary to determine the exact properties and effects of use.

General:
Rosewood is a tree native to the Amazon where the wood is harvested for use in furniture making and the oils extracted through steam distillation for use in perfumery, aromatherapy, and as a traditional supplement.

Sandalwood
Anaditam, Chandran, Chandana, Safed Chandan, Sandal Tree, Sandalwood, Santal, Tan

Xiang, White Sandalwood, Yellow Sandalwood, Yellow Saunders

Botanical Name:
Santalum album

Common Uses:
Acne, Natural Hair & Skin Care

Traditional Use:
Sandalwood is used as a toning astringent cleanser in natural hair & skin care products especially those designed to treat acne, skin inflammation, and dehydrated skin.

Part Used:
Wood   - Oil

Side Effects:
Sandalwood is not recommended for use other than aromatic by women who are pregnant or nursing.

Overuse of Sandalwood Oil may affect the kidneys.

Sandalwood may cause an allergic reaction to sandalwood including gastrointestinal upset, itching, and nausea.

Additional uses and side effects may exist but further research is necessary to determine the exact properties and effects of use.

General:
Sandalwood oil is extracted from the inner wood of the sandalwood tree. Sandalwood is a semi-parasitic tree that depends on other trees for nourishment early in its development. Sandalwood has been over harvested and presently considered an endangered botanical species. The oils are extracted through steam distillation for use in perfumery, aromatherapy, and supplemental treatments.

Sarsaparilla
Sarsaparilla, Smilax, Zarzaparilla

Botanical Name:
Smilax sarsaparilla

Common Uses:
Acne, Eczema, Natural Hair & Skin Care, PMS, Psoriasis

Traditional Use:
Sarsaparilla has anti-inflammatory and antibacterial properties that may make it a traditional skin wash treatment for certain types of acne, eczema, and psoriasis.

Sarsaparilla has traditionally been used to detoxify the body and reduce impurity related flare ups of conditions like acne, eczema, and psoriasis.

The phytochemicals in Sarsaparilla are believed to help sooth certain inflammatory conditions like acne, eczema, gout, and psoriasis by disabling certain bacterial components that build up in the blood and cause flare ups in each condition.

Sarsaparilla is sometimes used as an emulsifier in natural hair and skin care products.

Part Used:
Root

Side Effects:
Sarsaparilla is not recommended for use by women who are pregnant or nursing.

Sarsaparilla may cause asthma like symptoms in some people.

Over use or overdose of Sarsaparilla can cause kidney damage.

Additional uses and side effects may exist but further research is necessary to determine the exact properties and effects of use.

General:
Sarsaparilla is a woody climbing vine native to China, Central America & South America but cultivated in other regions. Sarsaparilla prefers rich, moist soil and part shade for optimal growth. Sarsaparilla is harvested in the late winter or early spring, dried and powdered for use in traditional supplements up to 3 times daily.

Sea Buckthorn
Common Names:
Argasse, Argousier, Chharma, Dhar Bu, Finbar, Grisset, Meerdorn, Oblepikha, Purging Thorn, Saddorn, Sea Buckthorn, Seedom, Star Bu, Tindved, Yellow Spine

Botanical Name:
Hippophae rhamnoides

Common Uses:
Acne, Anti-Aging, Damaged Skin, Eczema, Natural Skin Care, Seborrhea, Wounds

Traditional Use:
Sea buckthorn berry juice is rich in vitamins, phytosterols, anti-oxidants, and carotenoids. These give the oil potentially regenerative properties making it a traditional treatment for a variety of skin

disorders including acne, acute dryness, burns, eczema, and sun damage.

Sea buckthorn is used in natural skin care products to combat the formation of wrinkles and reverse premature aging of the skin caused by exposure to harsh environmental factors.

Sea Buckthorn oils have traditionally been used in topical preparations to speed healing in skin sores, ulcers, and wounds.

Part Used:
Berry, Juice, Seed, Oil

Side Effects:
Sea Buckthorn is not recommended for use by women who are pregnant or nursing.

Sea Buckthorn may reduce blood clotting action and is not recommended for use by people on blood thinning supplements, with a blood clotting disorder or who are undergoing surgery.

Undiluted sea buckthorn oil may stain the skin and other items.

Additional uses and side effects may exist but further research is necessary to determine the exact properties and effects of use.

General:
Sea Buckthorn is a hardy shrub native to China and Russia and grows naturally along the sea shore but can also be found in other habitats and regions. Sea Buckthorn is available in concentrates, juices, oils or powdered form and the traditional daily dosage is 10 grams.

Sea Grape
Bay Grape, Sea Grape

Botanical Name:
Coccoloba uvifera

Common Uses:
Acne, Wound Care

Traditional Use:
Sea Grape has been used as a traditional topical wash to help alleviate the severity of acne outbreaks.

Sea Grape has been used as a traditional topical preparation to speed healing and reduce the likelihood of infection in skin sores, ulcers, and wounds.

Part Used:

Bark – Gum, Leaf,

Side Effects:
Sea Grape is not recommended for use by women who are pregnant or nursing.

Sea Grape lowers blood sugar and should not be used without the advice of a physician or qualified herbalist.

Additional uses and side effects may exist but further research is necessary to determine the exact properties and effects of use.

General:
Sea Grape is a small tree native to the shoreline in Central America, South America and North America. The fruit is harvested for use as a cooked fruit and the bark, leaf, and fruit is harvested for use in supplement or topical decoctions.

Sesame
Botanical Name:
Sesamum indicum

Common Uses:
Natural Hair & Skin Care

Traditional Use:
Sesame seed oil is rich in vitamins A & E and contains essential proteins and anti-oxidants making it a frequently used carrier oil for natural hair & skin care products.

Part Used:
Seed, Seed Oil

Side Effects:
Sesame Seed is not recommended for use by women who are pregnant or nursing.

Additional uses and side effects may exist but further research is necessary to determine the exact properties and effects of use.

General:
Sesame is native to Africa and India but is naturalized to many tropical regions and is cultivated worldwide as a culinary seasoning, cooking oil, cosmetic ingredient, supplement or natural hair & skin care product ingredient.

Shatavari
Shatavari, Sathavari, Thaneevittan

Botanical Name:
Asparagus racemosus

Common Uses:
Acne

Traditional Use:
Shatavari has been used in topical washes to prevent certain types of bacterial acne and as a supplement to prevent hormonally stimulated acne outbreaks.

Part Used:
Whole

Side Effects:
Shatavari is not recommended for use by women who are pregnant or nursing.

Additional uses and side effects may exist but further research is necessary to determine the exact properties and effects of use.

General:
Shatavari is a species of asparagus native to India and cultivated in other regions where it is harvested for use as a food or for use as a traditional supplement treatment.

Soapwort
Bouncing Bet, Bruisewort, Fullers Herb, Red Soapwort

Botanical Name:
Saponaria officinalis

Common Uses:
Eczema, Natural Hair & Skin Care, Psoriasis

Traditional Use:
Soapwort is a common ingredient in cleaning products and skin care cleansers. Soapwort creates a mild lather on contact with Distilled Water and leaves behind a silky, slippery feeling.

Soapwort has traditionally been used as a topical preparation in the treatment of chronic skin conditions including eczema and psoriasis.

Part Used:
Leaf, Rhizome

Side Effects:
Soapwort is not recommended for use by women who are pregnant or nursing.

Soapwort is not recommended for use by people with inflammatory bowel disease or ulcers.

Soapwort is a purgative that may cause nausea, stomach irritation, and vomiting.

Soapwort is not recommended for internal use without the advice of a physician or qualified herbalist.

Soapwort may irritate the skin or mucus membranes.

Additional uses and side effects may exist but further research is necessary to determine the exact properties and effects of use.

General:
Soapwort is native to Asia, Europe and North America and can be found growing wild along roadsides and untended areas where the roots and leaves are harvested during the flowering season and used fresh or dried for use in traditional supplement teas or decoctions.

Spearmint
Curled Mint, Fresh Mint, Garden Mint, Green Mint, Lamb Mint, Mackerel Mint, Our Lady's Mint, Pahari Pudina, Sage of Bethlehem, Spearmint, Spire Mint, Yerba Buena

Botanical Name:
Mentha spicata

Common Uses:
Natural Skin Care

Traditional Use:
Spearmint is used in facial steam treatments and toning washes to cleanse & tighten pores.

Part Used:
Leaf, Oil

Side Effects:
Spearmint is not recommended for use by women who are pregnant or nursing.

General:
Spearmint is found in nearly every country of the world and is adapted to a variety of soil, sun, and Distilled Water conditions. It is considered an invasive weed by some. Spearmint oil is extracted from the flower, leaf, and stem harvested during the flowering season.

Speedwell
Gypsy weed, Speedwell, Veronica

Botanical Name:
Veronica officinalis

Common Uses:
Eczema, Psoriasis, Skin Irritation & Rash

Traditional Use:
Speedwell tea is traditionally used as a soothing wash to speed wound healing, calm itchy or irritated skin, and in treatments for eczema and psoriasis.

Part Used:
Flower, Leaf, Stem

Side Effects:
Speedwell is not recommended for use by women who are pregnant or nursing.

General:
Speedwell is native to Asia, Europe, and North America, Europe, and Asia and can be found growing in fields, ponds, and untended areas where it is harvested during the flowering season, dried, and powdered for use in traditional teas that have been given up to 3 times daily and externally as needed for relief from symptoms.

Spikenard
Fleabane, Indian Root, Old Man's Root, Pettymorell, Spignet, Spikenard

Botanical Name:
Aralia racemosa

Common Uses:
Contact Dermatitis, Natural Skin Care

Traditional Use:
Spikenard has been used as a traditional topical preparation to reduce inflammation and discomfort associated with skin conditions like contact dermatitis.

Spikenard is used in natural skin care products for its rejuvenating anti-inflammatory effects and is especially prized in treatments for mature skin.

Part Used:
Root

Side Effects:
Spikenard is not recommended for use by women who are pregnant or nursing.

Spikenard may cause skin irritation.

Additional uses and side effects may exist but further research is necessary to determine the exact properties and effects of use.

General:
Spikenard is native to the United States and can be found growing wild in open woods, thickets, and untended areas where it is harvested, dried, and powdered for use in traditional supplement infusions up to 3 times daily.

Sunflower
Adityabhakt, Corono Solis, Marigold of Peru, Sunflower

Botanical Name:
Helianthus annuus

Common Uses:
Natural Hair & Skin Care

Traditional Use:
Sunflower seed oil is an excellent source of Vitamin E and is used in natural cosmetic recipes to help combat wrinkles, promote a radiant glow, and to protect the hair & skin from UV rays and sun damage.

Part Used:
Leaf, Oil, Seed

Side Effects:
Sunflower is not recommended for use beyond dietary by women who are pregnant or nursing.

Sunflower may cause an allergic reaction in some people.

Sunflower may increase blood sugars.

Additional uses and side effects may exist but further research is necessary to determine the exact properties and effects of use.

General:
Sunflower is native to North America and is cultivated worldwide where the seeds are harvested for use as dietary oil or for use in supplement preparations. A traditional therapeutic dose of the oils in treating respiratory ailments is 15 drops 3 times daily. The leaves are harvested and dried for use as an infusion supplement.

Tamanu
Alexandrian Laurel, Indian Laurel, Kamani Punna, Palo Maria, Tamanu

Botanical Name:
Calophyllum inophyllum

Common Uses:
Acne, Eczema, Natural Skin Care, Psoriasis, Wound Care

Traditional Use:

Tamanu oil is rich oil with anti-inflammatory properties that is traditionally used in topical preparations to sooth symptoms and speed healing in conditions like acne, eczema, skin irritation, psoriasis, and wounds.

Tamanu oil is traditionally used to reduce scarring including acne scars, stretch marks.

Tamanu oil has been used as a traditional topical ointment or wash to speed healing of diabetic sores, fissures, chemical burns and herpes lesions.

Tamanu oil has significant antibacterial, antifungal, and antimicrobial qualities that make it a traditional treatment for a variety of infections like athlete's foot and staphylococcus.

Part Used:
Seed Oil

Side Effects:
Tamanu Oil is not recommended for use by women who are pregnant or nursing.

Tamanu Oil may cause dizziness, headache, and nausea.

General:
Tamanu is native to Africa, Asia and Australia but has been naturalized to other parts of the world as a fragrant ornamental. The seeds are harvested and the oils extracted by steam distillation for use in traditional topical and supplement preparations.

Tamarind
Imlee, Tamarind, Tintiri

Botanical Name:
Tamarindus indica

Common Uses:
Natural Skin Care, Wound Care

Traditional Use:
Tamarind oils have traditionally been used in natural skin care products as a tissue regeneration aide.

Tamarind has been used as a traditional poultice, ointment, or wash to reduce inflammation & infection while speeding healing in skin sores, ulcers, and wounds.

Part Used:
Fruit, Seed

Side Effects:

Tamarind is not recommended for use by women who are pregnant or nursing.

Additional uses and side effects may exist but further research is necessary to determine the exact properties and effects of use.

General:
Tamarind is a large evergreen native to Africa and has been naturalized to North & South America where the fruit is harvested when ripe for use as a food. The oil is extracted from the seed through steam distillation for use in topical preparations, cosmetics, and supplements.

Tea
Black Tea, Chinese Tea, English Tea, Green Tea, Tea

Botanical Name:
Camellia sinensis

Common Uses:
Eczema, Natural Skin Care - Skin Irritation

Traditional Use:
Brown tea has traditionally been used to reduce the number and severity of eczema outbreaks. Studies indicate that drinking 4 or more cups of oolong tea per day may help to reduce eczema.

Tea has analgesic, astringent, and stimulant properties that make it a nice additive in washes and ointments designed to treat sensitive, irritated, or problem skin and is traditionally used to provide faster healing of bruises, varicose veins, skin eruptions, and sun burns.

Part Used:
Leaves

Side Effects:
Tea is not recommended for use in women who are pregnant or nursing.

Tea is not recommended for use by people who have anemia, anxiety, bleeding disorders, diabetes, glaucoma, heart problems, high blood pressure, or osteoporosis.

Tea is not recommended for use in women who have a hormone sensitive condition like endometriosis, fibroids, and cancer.

Overdose of tea may cause confusion, convulsions, diarrhea, dizziness, headache, heartburn, irregular heartbeat, nervousness, sleep problems, tremor, and vomiting.

Green tea contains compounds that may make anti-coagulant drugs less effective.

Tea does contain caffeine and overuse may lead to anxiety, frequent urination, irritability, insomnia, restlessness, and upset stomach.

There have been reports of liver problems in some people taking a concentrated tea extract over an extended period of time.

Tea may be addictive.

Additional uses and side effects may exist but further research is necessary to determine the exact properties and effects of use.

General:
Black, brown and green teas come from the same plant and the difference in coloring is a result of a change in the way that the tea is handled during processing. The more extensive handling of black tea changes its phytochemicals make up making the green tea the more beneficial supplement. Brown Tea is only partially fermented while Black Tea is fully fermented and Green Tea is not fermented. Tea is typically brewed and consumed as a beverage but is available in extract form. Therapeutic doses are traditionally believed to be reached by drinking 1 teaspoon of green tea leaf in 1 cup boiling Distilled Water 5 times or more daily.

Thyme
French Thyme, Garden Thyme, Red Thyme, Rubbed Thyme, Spanish Thyme, Thyme, Tomillo, Van Ajwayan, White Thyme

Botanical Name:
Thymus vulgaris

Common Uses:
Acne, Wound Care

Traditional Use:
Thyme tea is often included in topical preparations to reduce the severity of acne outbreaks.

Part Used:
Flower, Leaf, Stem

Side Effects:
Thyme is not recommended for use by women who are pregnant or nursing.

Thyme can cause an allergic reaction in some people.

Thyme oil may elevate the blood pressure.

Overuse of thyme can effect the menstrual cycles in some women

The oils isolated from the plant can be toxic and should not be ingested but the herb itself is generally considered safe.

Additional uses and side effects may exist but further research is necessary to determine the exact properties and effects of use.

General:
Thyme is native to the Mediterranean but is cultivated in many areas of the world where it is harvested as a culinary seasoning and as a liquid extract for use in traditional supplements. The oils are extracted through steam distillation for use in aromatherapy. Red Thyme and White Thyme oil come from the same plant. The alteration in coloring is due to oxidation during the extraction and processing of the oils. Red Thyme oil contains stronger anti-septic properties and is traditionally used for disinfection. White Thyme oil has more of the impurities removed and tends to have a milder action making it preferred in many traditional treatments.

Turmeric
Curcuma, Halada, Haldi, Haridra, Indian Saffron, Nisha, Rajani, Turmeric, Yu Jin

Botanical Name:
Curcuma longa, Curcuma zedoaria

Common Uses:
Natural Skin Care, Wound Care

Traditional Use:
Turmeric supplements are used as a traditional supplement believed to work from the inside to help give skin a healthier, radiant glow.

Turmeric has traditionally been used to reduce the potential for infection in skin wounds & sores.

Part Used:
Rhizome, Underground Stems

Side Effects:
Turmeric is not recommended for use by women who are pregnant or nursing.

Turmeric may affect sugar levels do not use if you suffer from hyperglycemia or hypoglycemia.

Long term use or overdose of Turmeric may cause diarrhea, indigestion, or nausea in some people.

Turmeric is not for use by those with gall bladder disease.

Additional uses and side effects may exist but further research is necessary to determine the exact properties and effects of use.

General:
Turmeric is a shrub native to India and cultivated in China requiring warm temperatures and heavy moisture to survive. Turmeric is used in commercial and traditional supplements as a tea, powder, or liquid extract or made into a powder for topical applications.

Vanilla

Botanical Name:
Vanilla planifolia

Common Uses:
Natural Skin Care

Traditional Use:
Vanilla oil has been included in natural skin care treatments for its softening and smoothing action.

Part Used:
Bean

Side Effects:
Vanilla is not recommended for use beyond dietary by women who are pregnant or nursing.

Vanilla may cause skin irritation, headache and insomnia.

Additional uses and side effects may exist but further research is necessary to determine the exact properties and effects of use.

General:
Vanilla is commonly used as a flavoring around the world but has also been used in traditional supplements and aromatherapy treatments.

Violet

Sweet Violet, Viola, Violet, Wild Violet

Botanical Name:
Viola oderata

Common Uses:
Natural Skin Care, Wound Care

Traditional Use:

Violet is used in natural skin care preparations to sooth the skin, ease dryness, and leave a silky feeling.

Violet leaves have been used in traditional poultices and washes to reduce pain & inflammation while minimizing infection in wounds.

Part Used:
Whole

Side Effects:
Violet is not recommended for use by women who are pregnant or nursing.

Violet contains aspirin-like compounds and is not recommended for use by those who have sensitivity to aspirin, have a bleeding disorder, are on blood thinning medications, or in children's treatments.

Additional uses and side effects may exist but further research is necessary to determine the exact properties and effects of use.

General:
Violet is cultivated throughout the world and is most common within the Northern Hemisphere. Violet buds & leaves are eaten as a raw or cooked vegetable or as a flavorful thickening agent in soups & desserts. Violet leaf oil is extracted for use in perfumery and in aromatherapy treatments. The whole plant is harvested during flowering, and used fresh or dried & powdered for use in traditional infusions and supplements.

Walnut

Akschota, English Walnut, He Tao, Juglands, Juglandis, Nogal, Walnussblatter, Walnut

Botanical Name:
Juglans

Common Uses:
Acne, Eczema, Natural Hair & Skin Care, Skin Inflammation

Traditional Uses:
Walnut leaf is traditionally applied directly or included in topical ointments & washes to reduce inflammation, stop seepage, and speed healing in skin conditions like acne, eczema, inflammation, and ulcers.

Walnut hulls yield a dark brownish black dye colorant and are traditionally used to dye fabrics, as hair colorant, or as part of sunless tanning lotions.

Parts Used:
Nut, Shell – Hull

Side Effects:
Walnut is not recommended for use beyond dietary for women who are pregnant or nursing.

Walnut may cause softening of the stools, bloating and weight gain if it is used in excess.

Additional uses and side effects may exist but further research is necessary to determine the exact properties and effects of use.

General:
Walnut is the seed of the trees in the Jugulans family. Walnuts are eaten as a food and the nuts & hulls are used as a traditional supplement, cosmetic, and colorant.

Distilled Watercress
Agriao, Berros, Cresson, Indian Cress, Nasilord, Scruvy Grass, Tall Nasturtium, Distilled Watercress

Botanical Name:
Nasturtium officinale

Common Uses:
Acne

Traditional Use:
Distilled Watercress juice has been used as a traditional facial wash to reduce acne blemishes.

Part Used:
Whole

Side Effects:
Distilled Watercress is not recommended for women who are pregnant or nursing.

Distilled Watercress is not recommended for children.

Distilled Watercress may cause gastrointestinal upset including flatulence and nausea.

Additional uses and side effects may exist but further research is necessary to determine the exact properties and effects of use.

General:
Distilled Watercress is found in nearly every region of the world where it is harvested during the flowering season for use in salads or as a traditional supplement tea up to 4 times daily before meals.

Wheat

Botanical Name:
Triticum aestivum

Common Uses:
Contact Dermatitis, Damaged Skin, Eczema, Irritated Skin, Psoriasis

Traditional Use:
Wheat is traditionally added to baths & scrub bags to help alleviate itching associated with contact dermatitis, eczema, and psoriasis and to help heal damaged skin.

Side Effects:
Wheat is not recommended for use by women who are pregnant or nursing.

Additional uses and side effects may exist but further research is necessary to determine the exact properties and effects of use.

General:
Wheat is cultivated as a food crop in Asia, Europe and North America. Wheat is also used as a traditional supplement or topical preparation up to 2 times daily.

White Nettle
Archangel, Bee Nettle, Blind Nettle, Deaf Nettle, Dumb Nettle, Stingless Nettle, White Nettle

Botanical Name:
Lamium album

Common Uses:
Conluct Dermatitis, Skin Irritation & Inflammation

Traditional Use:
White Nettles have been incorporated into traditional washes to help alleviate skin irritation from contact dermatitis.

Part Used:
Flower, Leaf

Side Effects:
White Nettle is not recommended for use by women who are pregnant or nursing.

Additional uses and side effects may exist but further research is necessary to determine the exact properties and effects of use.

General:
White Nettle is native in Asia and Europe where the leaves are eaten as a raw or cooked vegetable. The flower and leaf have been harvested, dried, and powdered for use in traditional supplement

teas up to 3 times daily and for use as a topical poultice or wash.

Witch Hazel
Botanical Name:
Hamamelis virginiana

Common Uses:
Acne, Eczema, Natural Hair & Skin Care, Skin Rash, Psoriasis, Wound Care

Traditional Use:
The bark oil of witch hazel is combined with an alcohol base to create a soothing, astringent wash that works to sooth a variety of skin conditions from acne and eczema to varicose veins and eye puffiness.

Part Used:
Bark, Leaf, Oil

Side Effects:
Witch Hazel is not recommended for internal use by women who are pregnant or nursing.

Witch Hazel is not recommended for internal use. Internal use may cause constipation, gastrointestinal upset, liver problems and other side effects.

Additional uses and side effects may exist but further research is necessary to determine the exact properties and effects of use.

General:
Hamamelis virginiana is a species of Witch Hazel that is native to North America. The bark is harvested and distilled for use in traditional supplements, topical preparations, and commercial products.

Yarrow
Achilee, Milfoil, Nosebleed, Old Man's Pepper, Soldier's Woundwort, Staunchweed, Yarrow

Botanical Name:
Achillea millefolium

Common Uses:
Acne, Eczema, Scars, Wound Care

Traditional Use:
Yarrow has been used as a topical preparation to cleanse the skin and reduce the severity of acne outbreaks while also being taken as a supplement to cleanse the body of impurities helping to limit the number and severity of future outbreaks.

Yarrow is traditionally used to help heal inflamed cuts and wounds while minimizing scarring and soothing chronic conditions like eczema.

Part Used:
Flower, Leaf, Oil, Stem

Side Effects:
Yarrow is believed to have an abortifacient effect and is not recommended for use by women who are pregnant or nursing.

Yarrow may cause photosensitivity, allergic reactions, or skin irritation.

Yarrow is intended for short term use only.

Overuse of Yarrow can be toxic.

Overuse of Yarrow may cause headaches & dizziness.

General:
Yarrow is native to Asia and Europe and has been naturalized to North America growing wild in dry fields and untended areas. Yarrow is harvested, dried, and powdered for use in traditional supplement infusions given up to 4 times daily.

Yellow Dock
Acedera, Amalvelas, Broad Leaved Dock, Curled Dock, Field Sorrel, Narrow Dock, Rumex, Sheep Sorrel, Sour Dock, Yellow Dock

Botanical Name:
Rumex crispus

Common Uses:
Acne, Contact Dermatitis, Eczema, Skin Irritation, Poison Ivy, Psoriasis,

Traditional Use:
Yellow dock tea has traditionally been used as a supplement to help detoxify the body and treat chronic skin conditions and has also been incorporated into a wash to aid in reducing certain types of acne, eczema, psoriasis, and itchy contact dermatitis including poison ivy.

Part Used:
Root

Side Effects:
Yellow Dock is not recommended for use by women who are pregnant or nursing.

Overuse of Yellow Dock may cause potassium depletion.

Overuse of Yellow Dock may cause cramps, diarrhea, excessive urination, nausea, and skin irritation.

Overuse of Yellow Dock may irritate the mucus membranes and should not be used by people with ulcers.

Yellow dock may cause or aggravate kidney stones.

Yellow Dock may cause allergies in some people.

Yellow Dock may speed clotting.

Additional uses and side effects may exist but further research is necessary to determine the exact properties and effects of use.

General:
Yellow dock is native to Africa and Europe but has naturalized to other areas including the United States where some consider it an invasive weed. Yellow Dock prefers high moisture, porous soil and plenty of sunlight for optimal growth. The leaf is used as a salad food and the root is harvested in the spring, dried and powdered for use in traditional supplement teas and topical preparations.

GLOSSARY

Abortifacient – is a substance that is capable of inducing an abortion

Adoptogenic – is a substance that has a normalize effect against changes brought about by stressors

Alopecia – A condition where hair is lost or partially lost from a place where it normally grows also called baldness.

Amenorrhea – refers to the absence of normal menstruation.

Analgesic - is a pain-killing drug or medicine.

Anodyne - is a pain-killing drug or medicine.

Antibacterial – is a substance that is active against bacteria.

Anti-Convulsant – is a substance used to reduce or prevent convulsions.

Anti-Emetic – is a substance that reduces or prevents nausea or vomiting.

Anti-Fungal – is a substance that alleviates or prevents fungal infections.

Antihistamine - is a substance that inhibits the physiological effects of histamine. Histamine is the chemical released by the body during an allergic reaction.

Anti-Inflammatory – is a substance used to reduce inflammation.

Anti-Microbial- is a substance that kills or inhibits the growth of microorganisms

Anti-Oxidant – is a molecule that inhibits the oxidation of other molecules.

Anti-Periodic – is a substance used to treat malarial-type symptoms or to prevent the recurrence of malarial like symptoms.

Anti-Parasitic – is a substance used to treat or prevent parasitic infestations.

Anti-Septic – is a substance capable of preventing or treating infection by inhibiting the growth of microorganisms.

Anti-Spasmodic - is a substance that suppresses muscle spasms.

Anti-Tussive – is a substance used to suppress or relieve coughing.

Anti-Viral – is a substance that prevents or treats viral infections by killing a virus or that suppresses its ability to replicate.

Aphrodisiac – is a substance that stimulates sexual desire.

Aromatic – is a substance having a pleasant and distinctive smell that is used as a treatment.

Aroma Therapy – is the process of using an aromatic plant extract or essential oil to cause a physical or psychological effect in treatments.

Aspergillus - is a type of common mold that cause food spoilage and potentially disease.

Astringent - is a substance that causes the contraction of body tissues.

Botanical Name – is the Latin name give to a species of plant to distinguish it from other plants.

Bursitis – is a condition where there is inflammation in the bursa – elbow, knee, shoulder.

Cardiac – refers to the heart.

Carminative – is a substance that relieves flatulence.

Cathartic - is a purgative substance.

Chalagogue - is a substance that stimulates the secretion of bile from the gallbladder.

Coagulant - is a substance that causes blood to clot or coagulate

Colorant - is a substance that colors something usually food, cosmetics, or textile products.

Common Name – is the non-specific name used for everyday reference to a plant

Comminution – is the action of reducing a material or substance. When processing plants the act of reducing the size of the plant parts by cutting, grinding, or pounding

Conjunctivitis – is an infection or irritation causing inflammation, itching, and redness of the white part of the eye.

COPD – stands for Chronic Obstructive Pulmonary Disease, which is a disorder that involves constriction of the airways and difficulty breathing.

Decoction – is the result of concentration the essence of a substance or plant part by heating or boiling.

Demulcent – is a substance that soothes inflammation and protects irritated internal tissues.

Depurative – is a substance that facilitates the removal of impurities or cleansing of bodily fluids.

Detoxification - is the process of removing toxic substances or qualities from matter.

Diaphoretic – is a substance that induces perspiration.

Diosgenin – is a steroid compound used in the synthesis of steroid hormones.

Diuretic – is a substance causing increased passing of urine.

Dram – is a unit of measurement equaling approximately 1/16 of a dry weight ounce in US measurement 1/8 of a fluid ounce in Apothecary measurement.

Dysmenorrheal – refers to menstruation with excessive pain involving abdominal and lower back cramping.

Emetic - is a substance that causes vomiting.

Emmenagogue – is a substance that stimulates or increases menstrual flow.

Emollient – is a substance that has a softening or soothing affect on the skin.

Estrogenic – is a substance acting like, relating to, or caused by estrogen.

Expectorant – is a substance that promotes the secretion of mucus from the air passages.

Expression – is the process of forcibly separating liquids from solids.

Febrifuge – is a substance used to reduce fever.

Fluid extract – is a type of fluid-solid substance obtained from plant matter through Distilled Water or alcohol processing

Galactogogue - is a substance that stimulates milk secretion.

Glycosides – is a compound formed from a simple sugar and another compound by the replacement of a hydroxyl in the sugar molecules.

Gram-Positive Bacteria – is a class of bacterial that are stained dark blue or violet by gram staining including bacteria such as pneumococci, staphylococci, and streptococci.

Gram Negative Bacteria - A class of bacterial that do not retain the stain used in gram staining including bacteria such as e. coli, shingella, and salmonella.

Hallucinogenic – is a psychoactive substance capable of producing hallucinations or altered sensory experiences.

Hepatic – refers to being of or relating to the liver.

Hydration – is the process of combining with or giving Distilled Water.

Hypoallergenic – is a substance unlikely to cause an allergic reaction.

Hypoglycemic – is a condition indicated by low blood sugar.

Hypotensive – is a condition of abnormally low blood pressure.

Histamine – is the chemical released by the body during an allergic reaction.

Immuno-Stimulant - is a substance that stimulates the immune system to fight infection.

Infusion – Aqueous – is a drink or extract made by soaking plant parts in Distilled Water.

Infusion – Oil – is a drink, extract, or product made by soaking plant parts in oil.

Insecticide - Substance used for killing insects.

Interferon - is a protein released in response to a virus that has the ability to inhibit virus reproduction.

Laxative – is a substance that stimulates or facilitates evacuation of the bowels

Lipase – is an enzyme that facilitates the breakdown of fats to fatty acids and glycol to other alcohols.

Maceration – is the process of softening plant materials by soaking or steeping in a liquid. To separate the compounds by soaking or steeping

Menorrhagia – refers to abnormally heavy menstrual bleeding.

Menstruum - is a solvent or mix of solvents.

Microphage – is a cell found in the tissues or at the site of an infection that takes in foreign material.

Mordant – is a substance that combines with a dye or stain to fix the colorant into a material.

Muscle Relaxant – is a substance that reduces muscle tone or contractibility.

Narcotic – is a psychoactive substance affecting mood or behavior.

Nervine – is a psychoactive substance that calms the nerves.

Nutritive – is a substance that is nutritious or provides nourishment.

Percolation – is the extraction of soluble components by passing the liquid through a filtering medium.

Pharynx – is the membrane-lined cavity behind the nose and mouth that connects them to the esophagus.

Phytoestrogen – are compounds found in plants that can mimic the effects of estrogen.

Pleurae – is the membranes lining the thorax and enveloping the lungs.

Pleurisy – is an inflammation of the pleurae that causes pain when breathing.

Polysaccharide – is a carbohydrate that is a compound of sugar molecules bonded together.

Proof Spirit – is a mixture of alcohol and Distilled Water containing 50% alcohol by volume standard in the US.

Purgative – is a substance that is strongly laxative in effect.

Pulmonary – relates to the pulmonary system.

Phytosterol – is a group of naturally occurring steroid plant compounds.

Reparative – is a substance that helps to repair.

Rhinitis – is the inflammation of the mucus membrane of the nose.

Rubefacient – is a substance whose external application produces increased circulation or redness of the skin.

Saponins – is a class of steroid and terpenoid glycosides that are used in detergents and foams when shaken with Distilled Water.

Sciatica – refers to nerve pain caused by compression of a spinal nerve in the lower back that affects the back, hip, or leg.

Sedative – is a substance that causes a calming or sleep-inducing effect.

Squalene – is an oily liquid that is the precursor to sterols.

Sterols – is a naturally occurring unsaturated steroid alcohol.

Steroidal – relates to steroid hormones or their effects.

Stimulant – is a substance that raises levels of physiological or nervous activity in the body.

Styptic – is a substance that causes bleeding to stop.

Succus – refers to several liquids in the body commonly termed digestive juices but also to the juice of fresh plant material.

Tincture – is a substance made by dissolving plant materials in alcohol.

Vasodilator – is a substance that causes dilation of blood vessels.

Vermifuge – is a substance that destroys parasites.

Viscosity – is the resistance of a liquid to movement and flow.

www.ingramcontent.com/pod-product-compliance
Lightning Source LLC
Chambersburg PA
CBHW080103010626
45794CB00014B/3002